S0-BCL-329

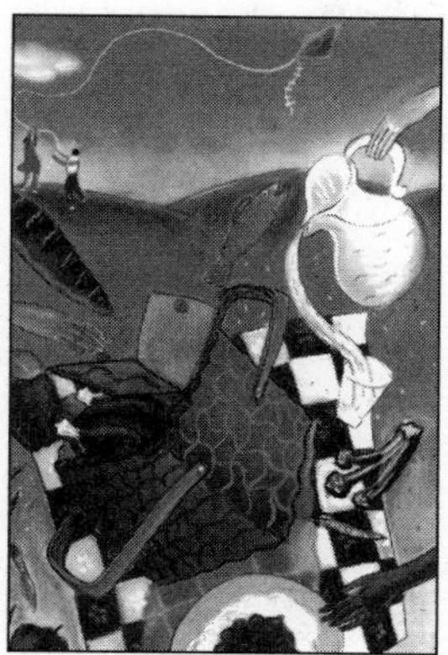

EAT FOR LIFE

The Food and Nutrition Board's Guide to Reducing Your Risk of Chronic Disease

Catherine E. Woteki, Ph.D., R.D.
and
Paul R. Thomas, Ed.D., R.D.
Editors

Committee on Diet and Health
Food and Nutrition Board

INSTITUTE OF MEDICINE

NATIONAL ACADEMY OF SCIENCES

NATIONAL ACADEMY PRESS
Washington, D.C. 1992

National Academy Press • 2101 Constitution Avenue, NW • Washington, DC 20418

NOTICE: The project that is the subject of this report was approved by the Governing Board of the National Research Council, whose members are drawn from the councils of the National Academy of Sciences, the National Academy of Engineering, and the Institute of Medicine. The members of the committee responsible for the report were chosen for their special competences and with regard for appropriate balance.

This report has been reviewed by a group other than the authors according to procedures approved by a Report Review Committee consisting of members of the National Academy of Sciences, the National Academy of Engineering, and the Institute of Medicine.

The Institute of Medicine was chartered in 1970 by the National Academy of Sciences to enlist distinguished members of the appropriate professions in the examination of policy matters pertaining to the health of the public. In this, the Institute acts under both the Academy's 1863 congressional charter responsibility to be an adviser to the federal government and its own initiative in identifying issues of medical care, research, and education.

The study summarized in this publication was supported by funds from the National Research Council Fund, the W.K. Kellogg Foundation, the Henry J. Kaiser Family Foundation, Pew Charitable Trusts, Fannie E. Rippel Foundation, and Occidental Petroleum Corporation. The Henry J. Kaiser Family Foundation supported the preparation of *Eat for Life.*

Library of Congress Cataloging-in-Publication Data

Eat for Life: the Food and Nutrition Board's guide to reducing your risk of chronic disease / Catherine E. Woteki and Paul R. Thomas, editors.

p. cm.

Includes bibliographical references and index.

ISBN 0-309-04049-3

1. Nutrition. 2. Chronic diseases—Prevention. I. Woteki, Catherine E. II. Thomas, Paul R., 1953- . III. Institute of Medicine (U.S.). Food and Nutrition Board.

RA784.E16 1992

613.2—dc20

91-37837

CIP

This book is printed on acid-free recycled stock that is made from 70% de-inked fiber of which 10% is postconsumer waste.

Printed in the United States of America

The serpent has been a symbol of long life, healing, and knowledge among almost all cultures and religions since the beginning of recorded history. The image adopted as a logotype by the Institute of Medicine is based on a relief carving from ancient Greece, now held by the Staatlichemuseen in Berlin.

Cover art by Mercedes McDonald

An Editorial Note

This book is the result of the work of many people and draws on more than a decade of study by the Food and Nutrition Board. It brings together the most current information on nutrition, gleaned from an exhaustive collection of data and professional literature that was reviewed and evaluated by nutrition scientists. The goal of all this effort: to determine whether diet has any effect on chronic disease.

When the Food and Nutrition Board began planning a study of what is known of diet and its relationship to chronic disease, three books were envisioned. The first was a comprehensive review and analysis of the scientific literature, which culminated in a massive volume published in 1989 under the title *Diet and Health.* That report makes specific recommendations on dietary changes to maintain health and prevent disease.

The second book to come from this study focused on implementing the dietary guidelines that emerged from the scientific review. If reducing the risk of chronic disease is a national health goal and if dietary modification is likely to help in achieving that goal, the Food and Nutrition Board reasoned that government, the private sector, health professionals, and educators would need a strategy for implementation. This book appeared in 1991 under the title *Improving America's Diet and Health: From Recommendations to Action.*

The present book, *Eat for Life,* is the final volume. Written for individuals and families interested in improving their health, it is a practical guide on how to incorporate the dietary guidelines into everyday life.

Special acknowledgment is owed to a small group of supporters who believed that this book could be completed successfully without compromising the material it covers. Joseph Alper, working from the voluminous original report, wrote the first draft of what was to become *Eat for Life.* Catherine Woteki, Paul Thomas, and editorial consultant Roseanne Price, together with members of the Food and Nutrition Board, revised and completed the manuscript in its present form. The many drafts of the manuscript were typed and proofread by Donna Thompson, Ute Hayman, Pamela Turner, and Marcia Lewis. The National Academy Press gave encouragement and technical assistance throughout the project.

The final success of this large endeavor involving so many people may never be known. We can only hope that it will be observed in the growing trend toward good health that emerges from knowledgeable individuals eating well.

C.E.W.
P.R.T.

CONTENTS

1 **Introduction** 1

Developing Nutritional Guidelines, 3
An Eating Pattern for Life—Not a "Diet" 5

2 **Guidelines for a New Eating Pattern** 9

The Nine Dietary Guidelines, 10
How These Guidelines Stack Up Against Others, 16
You Benefit, the Nation Benefits, 24
Dietary Terms, 27

3 **The Food We Eat** 33

What's in Food? 34
How Diet Has Changed Over Time, 53

4 **Diet and Chronic Disease in the United States** 57

Atherosclerosis (Hardening of the Arteries), 60
Heart Disease, 62
Peripheral Artery Disease, 63
Stroke, 64
High Blood Pressure (Hypertension), 65
Cancer, 67
Diabetes, 69
Obesity, 70
Osteoporosis, 75
Gallstones, 76
Cirrhosis of the Liver, 76
Dental Caries (Cavities), 77

5 **Calories, Energy Balance, and Chronic Diseases** 79

Fueling Up and Burning It Off, **80**
Weight and Chronic Illness, **81**
The Dieting Cycle, **84**

6 **Fats, Cholesterol, and Chronic Diseases** 87

Heart Disease, **87**
High Blood Pressure, **95**
Cancer, **96**
Other Chronic Degenerative Diseases, **98**
Children: A Special Case?, **98**

7 **Protein, Carbohydrates, and Chronic Diseases** 101

Protein, **102**
Carbohydrates, **103**
Fiber, **104**

8 **Vitamins, Minerals, and Chronic Diseases** 109

Vitamins, **110**
Minerals, **114**
Vitamin and Mineral Supplements, **119**

9 **Alcohol, Other Food Substances, and Chronic Diseases** 121

Alcohol, **122**
Coffee and Tea, **127**
Other Food Additives, **128**

10 **Making the Change to the New Eating Pattern** 131

What Foods Should I Eat? Some General Guidelines, **132**
Planning a Menu, **133**
Shopping, **136**

Cooking, **147**
Eating Out, **152**
Taking the Next Steps, **154**

APPENDIXES **157**

A U.S. Recommended Daily Allowances, **157**
B Resources, **161**
C Committee on Diet and Health and Food and Nutrition Board, **163**

Index **167**

EAT FOR LIFE

CHAPTER

1

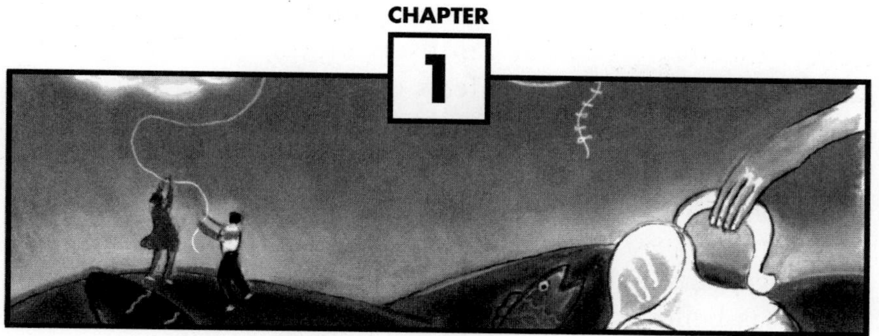

INTRODUCTION

The foods you choose to eat can have a direct impact on your ability to enjoy life to its fullest. Perhaps the most obvious positive effect of food is the pleasurable feeling you get from eating a good-tasting meal. It might be a plate of grilled chicken, corn-on-the-cob, fresh vine-ripened tomatoes, and a baked potato, or a steaming dish of spaghetti topped with a zesty tomato sauce.

Your diet can have long-term effects on your health as well. Diet plays a major role in promoting and maintaining good health, preventing some chronic diseases and treating others, and speeding recovery from injuries. In earlier times, diseases such as goiter and pellagra were relatively common—both are caused by nutritional deficiencies and cured by diets containing sufficient amounts of a particular nutrient. In the case of goiter, iodine is the missing nutrient; with pellagra it is mainly niacin, a B vitamin. These diseases are rare today in the United States because most Americans get enough of these essential nutrients in their diets.

Although it is unlikely that you or your family will ever suffer from an illness caused by pronounced dietary deficiency, the foods you eat can exert more subtle and, in the long run, no less harmful effects on your health. During the past few decades, scientists have identified several dietary factors that play important roles in the development of specific diseases. Diets high in certain types of fat, for example, appear to increase the risk of developing coronary heart disease and certain cancers, and, among susceptible people, too much salt in food is believed to increase the chances of developing hypertension (high blood pressure). Other scientific evidence suggests that the current average American diet—which is high in fatty foods and low in fruits and vegetables—can increase the risk of developing certain forms of cancer, especially cancers of the esophagus, colon (large bowel), prostate, and breast. Certain dietary patterns can increase the likelihood of dental caries (cavities). In addition, habitually eating more calories than the body uses for maintenance and physical activity produces obesity and increases the risk of several chronic diseases including noninsulin-dependent diabetes mellitus, a form of diabetes that does not usually require daily insulin injections but has many adverse complications and generally appears after age 40.

As the body of research on diet-disease connections has grown over the past half century, scientists, policymakers, officials of the food industry, consumer groups, and others have engaged in a debate about how much and what kind of evidence justifies giving dietary advice to the public. They have also argued about how best to control risk factors on which there is general agreement among scientists.

The central problem in this debate is one that characterizes all science: absolute proof is difficult to obtain. This is particularly true in a science such as nutrition, in which many factors—age, sex, genetics, social behavior, and cultural differences, for example—can play a role in what food we eat and how it affects our bodies.

Nevertheless, the strength of the evidence, the severity of the risk, and the ability of people to make informed choices can be used as a foundation for making public policy decisions on diet and health. Public information and education programs may be appropriate in some cases, and government regulation in others. For example, it might be sufficient to educate people against the potential hazard of eating too much fatty food, but the cancer-causing potential of aflatoxin (a toxin produced by a mold that grows on food) and the fact that it cannot be seen in food warrant government regulation to curtail aflatoxin contamination of peanuts, grains, and milk. Other criteria might come into play as well: the likelihood that a particular nutritional factor will trigger an increase in a chronic disease, the severity of that disease, the number of people likely to be affected, and estimates of whether people will change their eating habits in response to this risk.

DEVELOPING NUTRITIONAL GUIDELINES

To pin down diet-disease connections with an eye to providing the best possible dietary advice to the American public, the scientists of the Committee on Diet and Health of the Food and Nutrition Board (then under the National Research Council and since 1988 under the Institute of Medicine) reviewed thousands of pertinent studies. Most of the material in *Eat for Life* comes from the much larger volume *Diet and Health: Implications for Reducing Chronic Disease Risk* (National Academy Press, 1989), which was the primary result of that review.

The committee's charge was to determine what dietary constituents, if any, play a role in the occurrence of chronic diseases. Furthermore, the committee members were to recommend dietary changes that would promote longer, healthier lives for the general public of the United States by reducing the risk of chronic illness caused by current dietary practices.

Several other expert groups have also addressed the importance of dietary factors to the public's health (see chapter 2). But aside from the recent *Surgeon General's Report on Nutrition and Health* (U.S. Government Printing Office, 1988), these other groups have focused primarily on identifying dietary risk factors for single diseases.

The committee members decided that there is still much to be learned about diet and its role in chronic diseases. But they also concluded that it would be wrong to ignore the large body of existing evidence supporting a link between nutrition and chronic disease while waiting for absolute proof of the benefits that we as a nation, and as individuals, would gain from making certain changes in our diets.

After all their deliberations, the committee members decided that the overall evidence for a relationship between certain dietary patterns—a diet high in saturated fatty acids and total fat, for example—and chronic diseases–-such as heart attacks and certain cancers—supports three actions.

- First, they devised the nine dietary guidelines that are the basis of *Eat for Life.*
- Second, they concluded that there should be a comprehensive attempt to inform the public about the likelihood of certain risks and the possible benefits of dietary changes. That is the role of this book, as well as other efforts by the press, scientists, nutritionists, physicians, and public officials.
- Third, the committee strongly believes that government and the food industry should take steps to make it easier for us to change our diets. For example, beef producers should develop leaner meat that will make it easier to reduce the amount of fat in our diets. In the same vein, food processors should use less salt and saturated fat in their products, and fast-food chains should introduce lower-calorie and

lower-fat items to their menus. Government at all levels—federal, state, and local—should adopt policies and programs that promote the recommended changes and eating patterns.

AN EATING PATTERN FOR LIFE—NOT A "DIET"

The nine dietary guidelines devised by the committee can help reduce your risk of developing heart disease, hypertension, various forms of cancer, dental caries, obesity, noninsulin-dependent diabetes, osteoporosis, and chronic liver disease. These nine dietary guidelines are laid out in Table 1.1 and described in Chapter 2.

The thing to remember when you read these guidelines is that they are not the rules of a "diet." The eating pattern outlined in this book does not revolve around sacrifice. The eating pattern can work within the framework of any ethnic cuisine. It is not a list of foods you can and cannot eat, nor is it a series of menu plans to which you must adhere. Following this pattern is not expensive, and it may even lower your food bills. It is certainly not a complicated process that involves weighing food, dishing out exactly measured portions, or calculating the nutritional content of every meal you eat.

The nine dietary guidelines are just that: guidelines. They provide the foundation upon which you can build a sensible dietary pattern that suits your particular needs and tastes. These guidelines, in essence, form an eating pattern for life and provide you with a philosophy of eating that can guide you as you plan meals, cook, shop, and eat out.

Of course, following the guidelines may require you to make some changes in the way you eat. But those changes will be evolutionary, not revolutionary—you do not have to become a vegetarian, for instance, or eat exotic foods that you can find only at health food or specialty stores. You will learn to trim fat from the meat you eat—but you do not have to

TABLE 1.1 The nine dietary guidelines

1. Reduce total fat intake to 30 percent or less of your total calorie consumption. Reduce saturated fatty acid intake to less than 10 percent of calories. Reduce cholesterol intake to less than 300 milligrams (mg) daily.

2. Eat five or more servings of a combination of vegetables and fruits daily, especially green and yellow vegetables and citrus fruits. Also, increase your intake of starches and other complex carbohydrates by eating six or more daily servings of a combination of breads, cereals, and legumes.

3. Eat a reasonable amount of protein, maintaining your protein consumption at moderate levels.

4. Balance the amount of food you eat with the amount of exercise you get to maintain appropriate body weight.

5. It is not recommended that you drink alcohol. If you do drink alcoholic beverages, limit the amount you drink in a single day to no more than two cans of beer, two small glasses of wine, or two average cocktails. Pregnant women should avoid alcoholic beverages.

6. Limit the amount of salt (sodium chloride) that you eat to 6 grams (g) (slightly more than 1 teaspoon of salt) per day or less. Limit the use of salt in cooking and avoid adding it to food at the table. Salty foods, including highly processed salty foods, salt-preserved foods, and salt-pickled foods, should be eaten sparingly, if at all.

7. Maintain adequate calcium intake.

8. Avoid taking dietary supplements in excess of the U.S. Recommended Daily Allowances (U.S. RDAs) in any one day.

9. Maintain an optimal level of fluoride in your diet and particularly in the diets of your children when their baby and adult teeth are forming.

give up meat by any means, and you will eat more bread, pasta, potatoes, vegetables, and fruits.

This book is designed to help you and your family make beneficial changes in the way you eat with a minimum of effort and a maximum of effect. Along with each guideline in Chapter 2 is a short discussion on how it can help protect your health. The chapters that follow provide enough information about the links between diet and chronic illness to convince you of the need to alter your current eating pattern. And in Chapter 10 you will find practical advice on how to follow the guidelines easily in your everyday life and how to avoid common nutritional pitfalls.

In the end, you will probably be surprised at how easy it is to eat healthfully and to enjoy your meals today without compromising your health in the future.

CHAPTER

2

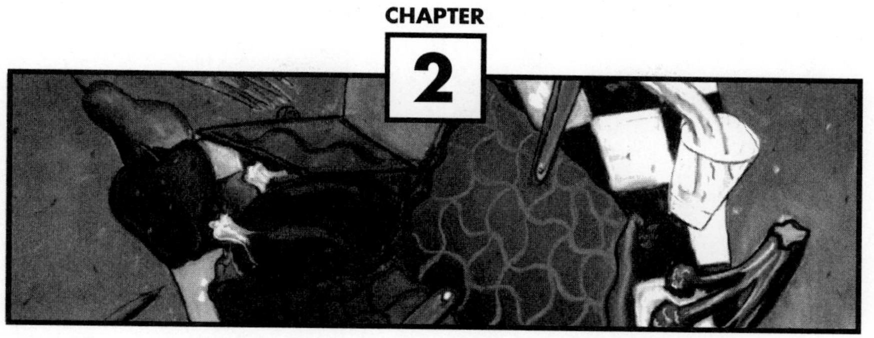

GUIDELINES FOR A NEW EATING PATTERN

In 1988 the surgeon general of the United States said, "For the two out of three adult Americans who do not smoke and do not drink excessively, one personal choice seems to influence long-term health prospects more than any other: what we eat." The scientific evidence linking diet and certain chronic diseases is strong and has been thoroughly documented in *Diet and Health*. This is not to say that diet is the whole story in causing these diseases. In fact, other aspects of lifestyle such as exercise, smoking, and drinking habits and various inherited, or genetic, factors also contribute to the risk of developing these illnesses. There is little you can do about the genes you inherit from your parents. However, you can modulate their effects through healthy lifestyle choices. Poor diet is one of several known disease-producing elements that you can change to benefit your own and your family's health.

The new eating pattern recommended by the Committee on Diet and Health consists of nine dietary guidelines. The guidelines were formulated to reduce the risk of not just one illness but an entire spectrum of chronic diseases. They also take into account whether making a dietary change to reduce the risk for one illness might raise the risk for another illness.

The guidelines are presented in a sequence that reflects their relative importance. For example, reducing fat intake has the highest priority because the scientific evidence concerning dietary fats and human health is strongest and the impact on your health is likely to be the greatest. In reading the guidelines, you may want to refer to the definitions of certain nutritional terms given on pages 27 through 31. These terms are explained in greater detail in the chapters to come.

THE NINE DIETARY GUIDELINES

1. Reduce total fat intake to 30 percent or less of your total calorie consumption. Reduce saturated fatty acid intake to less than 10 percent of calories. Reduce cholesterol intake to less than 300 milligrams (mg) daily.

Americans' diets average about 36 percent of their calories from fat and 13 percent of calories from saturated fatty acids. But a large and convincing amount of evidence shows that diets high in saturated fatty acids and cholesterol are associated with increased levels of cholesterol in the blood stream (serum cholesterol) and the consequent buildup of fatty plaque on the walls of blood vessels. Plaque causes arteries to become narrowed, less elastic, and eventually obstructed and is a cause of heart attacks and strokes.

The biggest contributors of saturated fatty acids to Americans' diets are dairy and meat products. Coconut, palm, and palm kernel oils contain higher levels of saturated fatty acids than other vegetable oils, but these oils are not usually eaten in large quantities by Americans. The major food groups providing dietary cholesterol are meat, poultry, and fish; egg yolks (which account for 39 percent of the cholesterol in the food supply); and, to a lesser extent, dairy products.

Evidence from many studies also links high-fat diets to a high incidence of some types of cancer, particularly cancer of the colon, prostate, and possibly breast. In addition, some studies suggest that high-fat diets may lead to obesity.

Thus this guideline is based on a wealth of scientific evidence. Reducing the amount of total fat and saturated fatty acids that you eat is likely to lower your risk of atherosclerotic cardiovascular disease, cancers of the colon and prostate, and possibly breast cancer and obesity.

You can reduce your intake of fat and cholesterol by substituting fish, poultry without skin, lean meats, and low-fat or nonfat dairy products for fatty meats and whole-milk dairy products; by including more vegetables, fruits, cereals, and legumes in your diet; and by limiting the amounts of oils, fats, egg yolks, fried foods, and other fatty foods that you eat.

You might be concerned that by eating less fatty meat and whole-milk dairy products you may not be getting enough iron and calcium. The Committee on Diet and Health found that you can safely reduce fat intake to 30 percent or less of your daily calories without risk of nutrient deficiency because most nutrients are found in the lean part of meat and the nonfat part of dairy products. In addition, children can still get enough calories in a diet containing 30 percent of calories from fat to ensure optimal growth and development. To accomplish this fat intake reduction, you will need to pick lean cuts of meat and low-fat dairy products, keep portion sizes of meat to 3 ounces (6 ounces a day), trim the visible fat, and cook lean.

One more word on this guideline: 30 percent of calories from total fat, 10 percent saturated fatty acids, and 300 mg of cholesterol per day are upper limits. Evidence suggests that if adults reduce those levels further, they may gain even greater health benefits. However, you should not attempt to eliminate all fat, especially in the diets of young children, because some fatty acids are essential for adequate growth and development.

2. Eat five or more servings of a combination of vegetables and fruits daily, especially green and yellow vegetables and citrus fruits. Also, increase your intake of starches and other complex carbohydrates by eating six or more daily servings of a combination of breads, cereals, and legumes.

An average serving is equal to one-half cup for most raw or cooked vegetables and fruits, one medium piece of fresh fruit, one-half cup dry or cooked cereal, one slice of bread, or one roll or muffin.

The scientific evidence suggests that carbohydrates should account for more than 55 percent of your daily calories (compared to about 45 percent in the average American diet today). Many of the foods listed above are rich in complex carbohydrates but low in fat. Thus they are good substitutes for fatty foods. These foods are also good sources of several vitamins, minerals, and dietary fiber.

Studies in various parts of the world indicate that people who habitually consume a diet high in plant foods have low rates of atherosclerotic cardiovascular disease, probably because such diets are usually low in animal fat and cholesterol. The evidence also reveals a link between lower susceptibility to cancers of the lung, stomach, and colon and frequent consumption of vegetables and fruits, particularly citrus fruits, green vegetables, and yellow vegetables, such as carrots and sweet potatoes.

Stroke is especially common among blacks and older people of all races. A diet high in potassium and low in sodium may contribute to reduced risk of stroke. Since vegetables and fruits are good sources of potassium, eating the recommended five servings per day of fruits and vegetables can help to lower your risk of stroke.

3. Eat a reasonable amount of protein, maintaining your protein consumption at moderate levels.

Protein-containing foods are important sources of amino acids. However, there are no known benefits and possibly some risks in eating diets with a high meat content. Therefore you should not increase your protein intake to compensate for the loss of calories that will result from eating less fat. In fact, most adults already eat considerably more protein than they need. Thus you should consume lean meat, and you may need to select smaller and fewer portions than is now customary in the American diet. One suggestion is to limit meat to 6 ounces a day; a 3-ounce portion of meat is about the size of a deck of cards.

4. Balance the amount of food you eat with the amount of exercise you get to maintain appropriate body weight.

Excess weight is associated with an increased risk of several chronic disorders, including noninsulin-dependent diabetes, high blood pressure, coronary heart disease, gallbladder disease, osteoarthritis, and endometrial cancer. The risks decline following a *sustained* reduction in weight.

The solution to being overweight is not merely reducing calories. In the United States and other Western societies, average body weight is increasing while the overall amount of calories consumed is dropping. The discrepancy between the high prevalence of excess weight and the low energy intake is probably attributable to low levels of physical activity. Thus we as a nation need to exercise more. Moderate, regular physical activity should be a part of everyone's regular routine.

5. It is not recommended that you drink alcohol. If you do drink alcoholic beverages, limit the amount you drink in a single day to no more than two cans of beer, two small glasses of wine, or two average cocktails. Pregnant women should avoid alcoholic beverages.

Several studies have shown that drinking moderate amounts of alcohol (one to two drinks per day) may reduce the risk of coronary heart disease, but drinking alcoholic beverages is not recommended as a way to prevent heart disease.

First and foremost is the risk of alcohol addiction. In addition, drinking too much increases your risk of developing heart disease, high blood pressure, chronic liver disease, some forms of cancer, neurological diseases, nutritional deficiencies, and many other disorders.

Even moderate drinking carries some risks in circumstances that require good coordination and judgment—driving and working around machinery, for example. Furthermore, pregnant women, as well as women who are attempting to become pregnant, should avoid alcoholic beverages because of the risk of damage to the fetus. No safe level of alcohol intake during pregnancy has been established.

6. Limit the amount of salt (sodium chloride) that you eat to 6 grams (g) (slightly more than 1 teaspoon of salt) per day or less. Limit the use of salt in cooking and avoid adding it to food at the table. Salty foods, including highly processed salty foods, salt-preserved foods, and salt-pickled foods, should be eaten sparingly, if at all.

Because food labels usually state the amount of sodium in a product rather than salt, it should be noted that 6 g of salt equals about 2400 mg of sodium.

In parts of the world where people eat more than 6 g of salt per day, hypertension is common. Many Americans regularly eat more than 6 g of salt per day, and this may be one reason that high blood pressure is fairly common in the United States. There is evidence, too, that reducing salt intake further, to less then 4.5 g per day, would have an even greater impact on reducing the risk of hypertension, but 6 g per day is a good start.

There is also consistent evidence that excessive consumption of salt-preserved or salt-pickled foods frequently increases the risk of stomach cancer. Some evidence links salt intake itself to stomach cancer, although it is not as persuasive as the connection between high salt intake and hypertension.

7. Maintain adequate calcium intake.

Calcium is an essential nutrient, necessary for proper growth and bone development. Certain groups of people, especially women and teenagers, need to choose their food carefully to obtain enough calcium from their diets. Getting enough calcium during the years when bones are growing will ensure that peak bone mass is achieved. This will decrease the risk of osteoporosis in later life. The best way to get enough calcium is to eat low-fat or nonfat milk and milk products and dark-green vegetables, all of which are rich in calcium. If you follow this advice, you do not need to take dietary calcium supplements.

8. Avoid taking dietary supplements in excess of the U.S. Recommended Daily Allowances (U.S. RDAs) in any one day.

Many people in the United States take a vitamin or mineral supplement daily. But except for people with special circumstances, supplements are not really necessary. The American Dietetic Association, American Institute of Nutrition, American Society for Clinical Nutrition, and the National Council Against Health Fraud have described categories of people who may need supplements. These include women with excessive menstrual bleeding; women who are pregnant or breastfeeding; people with very low caloric intakes; some vegetarians; newborns; and people with certain disorders or diseases or who are taking medications that may interfere with nutrient intake, digestion, absorption, metabolism, or excretion. The organizations recommend that individuals see their doctors or a registered dietitian to determine whether supplements are needed. For healthy people eating a varied diet, a single daily dose of a multiple vitamin-mineral supplement containing 100 percent of the U.S. RDAs is not known to be harmful or beneficial. High-potency vitamin-mineral supplements and other supplements such as protein powders, single amino acids, fiber, and lecithin, have no known health benefits. Large dose supplements may, in fact, be detrimental to your health. The best way to get all the nutrients you need is to eat a variety of foods.

9. Maintain an optimal level of fluoride in your diet and particularly in the diets of your children when their baby and adult teeth are forming.

The evidence is striking—drinking fluoridated water significantly reduces the risk of dental caries in people of all ages, although it is particularly effective in children when their teeth are growing. There is no evidence that fluoride, at the concentrations used in drinking water, has any adverse effects on health. If the water in your area is not fluoridated at the proper level (0.7 to 1.2 parts per million), you should use a dietary fluoride supplement recommended by the American Dental Association under the direction of your doctor or dentist. To find out if your community's water supply is fluoridated, contact the water authority of the local public works administration.

HOW THESE GUIDELINES STACK UP AGAINST OTHERS

In the recent history of dietary recommendations for overall health, an expert group from Sweden, Norway, and Finland was among the first to propose in 1968 that the general public should not eat too many calories; should reduce its fat consumption from 40 percent to between 25 and 30 percent of calories; should reduce the amount of saturated fatty acids and increase the amount of polyunsaturated fatty acids in the diet; should reduce consumption of sugar and sugar-containing foods; and should increase consumption of vegetables, potatoes, skim milk, fish, lean meat, and cereal products. Sounds familiar, doesn't it?

From the time of the Scandinavian report to this one, seven groups in the United States have proposed dietary guidelines that aim at preventing a range of diseases. These recommendations are shown in Table 2.1.

In addition, many expert groups have focused on specific diseases. These recommendations are shown in Table 2.2. In the early 1960s, the American Heart Association became the first U.S. organization to recommend dietary modifications for reducing heart disease. The National Cancer Institute issued its first set of dietary guidelines for cancer prevention in 1979, and the American Diabetes Association contributed dietary recommendations for avoiding noninsulin-dependent diabetes in 1987.

The two tables show that there is general agreement among the many sets of recommendations. The few differences of opinion that do exist stem largely from incomplete evidence on the link between diet and chronic diseases. Most of the recommendations deal with the type and amount of fat and cholesterol; complex carbohydrates, fiber, and sugars; sodium, salt, or salty foods; alcoholic beverages; and variety in the diet, as well as body weight and exercise. Some also address avoiding toxic substances, and two reports focus specifically on dietary supplements.

A few of the recommendations specify quantities of nutrients—percentage of calories from fat or grams of salt per day, for example. Others are more general in nature, suggesting that people should eat more of or avoid a particular dietary component.

In general, it is striking how much the recommendations from different sources agree. For example, because obesity is a major contributor to several chronic diseases, most expert panels have recommended maintenance of an appropriate body weight; some have even proposed height/weight tables such as the ones used by the life insurance industry (see Chapter 4).

The *Eat for Life* guidelines go along with the recommendation to keep to an appropriate weight, but here it is emphasized that you should balance your physical activity

TABLE 2.1 Dietary Recommendations to the U.S. Public, 1977 to 1990

	Maintain Appropriate Body Weight, Exercise	Limit or Reduce Total Fat (% kcal)	Reduce Saturated Fatty Acids (% kcal)	Increase Polyunsaturated Fatty Acids (% kcal)	Limit Cholesterol (mg/day)	Limit Simple Sugars
U.S. Senate (1977)	Yes	27-33	Yes	Yes	250-350	Yes
Council on Scientific Affairs (AMA) (1979)	Yes	No	No	No	No	Yes
DHEW (1979)	Yes	Yes	Yes	NS	Yes	Yes
NRC (1980)	Yes	For weight reduction only	No	No	No	For weight reduction only
USDA/DHHS (1980, 1985)	Yes	Yes	Yes	No	Yes	Yes
DHHS (1988)	Yes	Yes	Yes	No	Yes	Yes
USDA/DHHS (1990)	Yes	Yes	Yes	No	Yes	Yes

NOTE: NC = No comment; NS = Not specified. AMA = American Medical Association; DHEW = Department of Health, Education, and Welfare; NRC = National Research Council; USDA = U.S. Department of Agriculture; DHHS = U.S. Department of Health and Human Services.

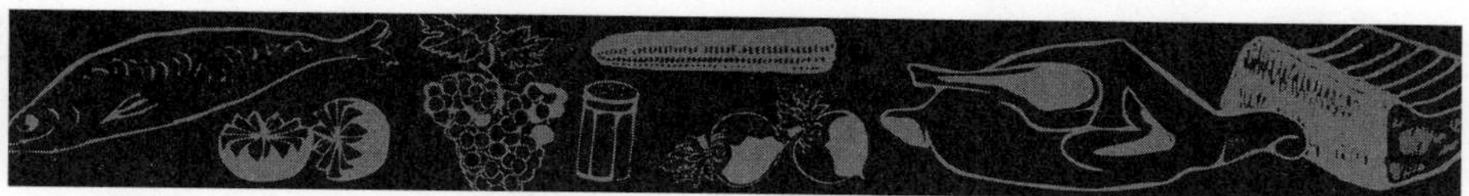

Increase Complex Carbohydrates (% kcal from *total* carbohydrates)	Increase Fiber	Restrict Sodium Chloride (g)	Moderate Alcohol Intake	Other Recommendations
Yes	Yes	8	Yes	Reduce additives and processed foods
NC	NC	12	Yes	Consider high-risk groups
Yes	NS	Yes	Yes	More fish, poultry, legumes; less red meat
No	No	3-8	For weight reduction only	Variety in diet; consider high-risk groups
Eat adequate starch and fiber		Yes	Yes	Variety in diet; consider high-risk groups
Yes	Yes	Yes	Yes	Fluoridation of water; adolescent girls and women increase intake of calcium-rich foods; children, adolescents, and women of child-bearing age increase intake of iron-rich foods
Choose diet with plenty of vegetables, fruits, and grain products		Yes	Yes	Variety in diet

SOURCE: National Research Council. 1989. *Diet and Health: Implications for Reducing Chronic Disease Risk.* National Academy Press, Washington, D.C.

TABLE 2.2 Dietary Recommendations to Reduce Risk of Specific Chronic Diseases

	Maintain Appropriate Body Weight, Exercise	Limit or Reduce Total Fat (% kcal)	Reduce Saturated Fatty Acids (% kcal)	Increase Polyunsaturated Fatty Acids (% kcal)	Limit Cholesterol (mg/day)	Limit Simple Sugars
Osteoporosis						
NIH (1984)	Exercise	NC	NC	NC	NC	NC
Diabetes						
ADA (1987)	Yes	<30	Yes	No	<300	Yes
Heart Disease						
Inter-Society Commission for Heart Disease Resources (1984)	Yes	<30	8	10	<250	NC
NIH (1985)	Yes	<30	<10	Up to 10	250-300	[a]
AHA (1988)	Yes	<30	<10	Up to 10	<300	NS
Cancer						
NRC (1982)	NC	~30	Yes	No	NC	NC
ACS (1984)	Yes	~30	Yes	No	NC	NC
NCI (1987)	Yes	Yes	Yes	No	NC	NC

[a]Endorsed recommendations of AHA (1982) and Inter-Society Commission for Heart Disease Resources (1984)

NOTE: NC = No comment; NS = Not specified. ADA = American Diabetes Association; NIH = National Institutes of Health; AHA = American Heart Association;

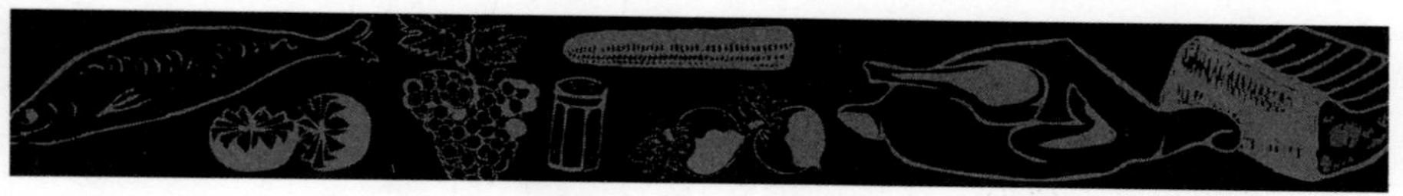

Increase Complex Carbohydrates (% kcal from *total* carbohydrates)	Increase Fiber	Restrict Sodium Chloride (g)	Moderate Alcohol Intake	Other Recommendations
NC	NC	NC	NC	Raise calcium to 1000 mg/day (premenopausal), 1500 mg/day (post-menopausal); use calcium supplements if needed; use vitamin D for calcium absorption
55-60	Yes	Yes	Yes	Nonnutritive sweeteners permitted but not recommended; limit protein to RDA level; avoid supplements except in special cases
Increase to make up caloric deficit	NC	5 g/day	NC	NS
a	*a*	NC	NC	Specific recommendations for high-risk groups; also physicians, public, and food industry
≥50	NS	≤3 g/day of sodium	1-2 oz ethanol/day	Protein to make up remainder of calories; wide variety of foods
Through whole grains, fruits, and vegetables	NS	By limiting intake of salt-cured, pickled, smoked foods	Yes	Emphasize fruits and vegetables; avoid high doses of supplements; pay attention to cooking methods
Same as NRC (1982)	Yes	Same as NRC (1982)	Yes	Same as NRC (1982)
Yes, more whole grains, fruits, and vegetables	To 20-35 g/day	NC	Yes	Variety in diet; avoid fiber supplements

NRC = National Research Council; ACS = American Cancer Society; NCI = National Cancer Institute.

SOURCE: National Research Council. 1989. *Diet and Health: Implications for Reducing Chronic Disease Risk*. National Academy Press, Washington, D.C.

with the amount of food you eat to avoid obesity. Merely watching your calories is not the best approach to weight control. And along with the American Dietetic Association, the committee recommends that you avoid gaining and losing weight repeatedly.

Perhaps the most common and consistent recommendation in these reports is to limit how much fat you eat. In most cases, the experts agree that fat should account for no more than 30 percent of your total calories. Most experts also suggest reducing the amount of saturated fatty acids you eat to less than 10 percent of total calories.

There is less agreement on recommendations concerning cholesterol in the diet. Most organizations advise that you eat less than 300 mg of cholesterol a day. Lower goals may be beyond the reach of the typical U.S. adult and thus may discourage people from trying to meet them.

The committee goes along with the consensus on fats and cholesterol. But you should keep one thing in mind: the dietary pattern recommended in *Eat for Life* is only moderately low in fat. The scientific evidence suggests that adults may achieve additional health benefits by cutting even more fat, saturated fatty acids, and cholesterol from their diets.

Most groups also advise that you should eat more complex carbohydrates to replace the calories from the fat that you cut from your diet. Some organizations have also singled out dietary fiber as something you should eat more of or refined sugar as a substance you should eat less of.

Eat for Life agrees with these other reports in suggesting that you eat more vegetables, grains, and legumes as sources of complex carbohydrates. However, this book also tells you how many servings per day of these foods you should eat. But unlike some guidelines, the ones in *Eat for Life* do not specifically include one to increase the amount of dietary fiber you eat. The Committee on Diet and Health believes that the evidence supports a recommendation to eat more fiber-rich foods (fruits, vegetables, cereals, and grains) rather than eating more fiber per se. Nevertheless, following the guidelines in this book will provide you with more than enough fiber.

Few reports deal with how much protein you should eat, although some say you should eat less meat and more vegetable products. If you adopt the *Eat for Life* pattern, the amount of protein you eat will remain about constant or perhaps drop some. The *Eat for Life* guidelines on salt and alcohol are also consistent with those of other groups.

Other reports have addressed specifically the need for vitamins and minerals. If you follow the guidelines in this book you will have no worries about getting the full range of nutrients in the amounts that you need. Like other books, *Eat for Life* suggests that you avoid taking dietary supplements in excess of the U.S. RDAs in any one day.

Eat for Life—and its parent report *Diet and Health*—differs from these other reports primarily in scope. This report looks at the effect of diet on a whole spectrum of chronic diseases influenced by diet. Developing the guidelines in *Eat for Life* required the committee members to analyze and compare recommendations that others have made for individual diseases to ensure that a guideline to reduce the risk of one chronic disease might not inadvertently increase the risk of another. By taking such a wide-ranging look at diet and health, the guidelines in *Eat for Life* can take into account competing risks from different dietary components and food groups. For example, recommendations to increase calcium intake to provide possible protection against osteoporosis might conflict with recommendations for heart disease prevention, because milk and milk products—the major source of calcium in the U.S. diet—are also major sources of saturated fatty acids. Therefore a guideline whose goal was to both maintain adequate bone mass and prevent heart disease would have to stress low-fat or nonfat dairy products.

YOU BENEFIT, THE NATION BENEFITS

There are two approaches to reducing dietary risk factors for chronic disease. The first is to make recommendations for individuals who are at higher risk, an approach that requires identifying and treating those who stand a good chance of developing a chronic illness. For example, high blood pressure, obesity, high serum cholesterol levels, atherosclerosis, and certain cancers appear to occur more frequently in particular families. The second method is to make recommendations aimed at the general public, hoping in the process to help everyone who might be at some risk for developing chronic diseases.

In a perfect world, dietary guidelines would be tailored for each person's individual biochemical needs. Such guidelines would account for a person's age, sex, heredity, body build, occupation, and other special conditions, such as pregnancy or illness. These would be ideal because each person is unique.

For conditions such as high blood pressure or elevated serum cholesterol levels, physicians can identify those of us at risk—in this case for stroke and heart disease, respectively—by using simple diagnostic tests. For other conditions where specific tests are lacking—such as breast cancer—a strong family history of the disease may suggest that special preventive approaches are needed. But for the most part, it is usually not feasible to identify people at high risk for a disease or to screen the entire population, and so dietary guidelines must apply to the general public.

By reaching a broader group of people, dietary recommendations aimed at reducing the risk in the general population can provide major health benefits for the nation. One study estimated that making changes similar to those in the *Eat for Life* guidelines could prevent more than 100,000 deaths annually from coronary heart disease, the nation's leading killer. In fact, the death rate for heart disease, which claims nearly a million lives a year, has already declined 33 percent since 1970, and a large part of this decline is related to the dietary changes some people have made already. You do not have to have remarkably high serum cholesterol levels to benefit from these guidelines, either. The vast majority of people who die from cardiovascular diseases have only moderately high total serum cholesterol levels: less than 240 milligrams per deciliter (mg/dl) but greater than 200 mg/dl. For moderately elevated total serum cholesterol, every 1 percent reduction in total serum cholesterol level in the U.S. population reduces the risk of coronary heart disease by 2 to 3 percent.

Incidences of other diseases would be reduced as well. Evidence on the connection between diet and cancer suggests that following these guidelines could eventually result in as much as a 35 percent reduction in cancer deaths in the United States. Hypertension affects an estimated 60 million people in the United States. If lowering salt intake cut that number by as little as 10 percent, that would mean 6 million more people a year would have less risk of stroke and heart disease.

Furthermore, although genetic factors can affect an individual's susceptibility to diseases, these inherited factors are not the entire story. Witness the fact that immigrants tend to acquire the disease rates of their adoptive countries, presumably because they adopt the lifestyle and the diet of the natives.

Therefore the guidelines in *Eat for Life* are for everyone except infants and children under 2 years to follow. Children, of course, will eat smaller serving sizes than the ones recommended for adults. Adhering to these guidelines should reduce the risk of chronic disease for everyone in the population—some of us will benefit more, but all of us are likely to benefit to some degree.

It is important to note, however, that even though the guidelines are written for the general public, the goals expressed are goals for the individual, not the general population. For example, the guideline that states that you should get less than 10 percent of your total calories from saturated fatty acids comes from evidence that average levels of total serum cholesterol are low in cultures in which the average consumption of saturated fatty acids is less than 10 percent of calories and that these cultures are relatively free of heart disease. However, the way the guideline is stated here is that each one of us—not just the nation as an average—should lower the amount of saturated fatty acids we eat to less than 10 percent.

Figure 2.1 illustrates this difference using serum cholesterol levels as the example. The dashed line shows serum cholesterol levels in a particular population ranging from 140 mg/dl to 260 mg/dl, with an overall average of 200 mg/dl. In that group of people, heart attacks are not common, but those few people who do have heart attacks tend to be those with cholesterol levels above 200 mg/dl.

The solid line indicates a population in which almost everyone has serum cholesterol levels below 200 mg/dl. As a result, the average cholesterol level for the whole population

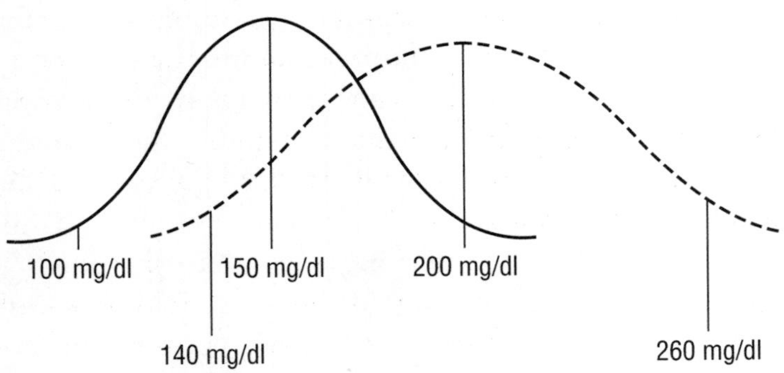

FIGURE 2.1 Hypothetical distributions of serum total cholesterol levels in a population that has achieved a public health goal of 200 mg/dl (dashed line) or a goal that all individuals lower their serum cholesterol to 200 mg/dl or less (solid line). For the lower goal, the range of cholesterol levels is assumed to be narrower. SOURCE: National Research Council. 1989. *Diet and Health: Implications for Reducing Chronic Disease Risk*. National Academy Press, Washington, D.C.

is approximately 150 mg/dl. All the members of this population are at low risk for heart disease, and although the level of heart disease is low in the population represented by the dotted line, it would be even lower in the population represented by the solid line.

There is another way to think about these guidelines and their possible positive effect on your health. Chances are good that your parents had you vaccinated against polio. The chances were small that you would ever catch polio, and even if you had caught polio your genetic makeup might have spared you permanent disability. Nevertheless, your parents decided to protect you against polio because even though the risk was small, the consequences could have been devastating.

The same is true here, except that the risk of developing cancer, coronary heart disease, stroke, or other chronic illness is much higher than that of catching polio. Each of us has a different genetic makeup that gives us different susceptibilities to chronic diseases; for example, some may be at high risk for cancer of the colon but at lower risk for cardiovascular disease, and vice versa. Because we are not able at this stage to distinguish who is at high or low risk for either of these diseases, we have to assume that everyone eating high levels of fat is at high risk. So until medical science can screen each and every one of us for our susceptibility to all chronic diseases, it would be wise for all of us to follow the dietary guidelines in *Eat for Life*.

DIETARY TERMS

Basic nutrition is covered more completely in Chapter 3, but a brief introduction here will make it easier to understand the guidelines.

Fats (also called **lipids**) are a large family of compounds that do not mix with water. Lard, butter, margarine, shortening, and cooking oil are almost pure fat; meat, dairy products, chocolate, cakes and cookies, nuts, and a few fruits and vegetables contain significant amounts of fat. Fats are important sources of energy in the diet.

Fatty acids are the major components of fats. They come in three basic types: **saturated fatty acids, monounsaturated fatty acids,** and **polyunsaturated fatty acids.** Saturated fatty acids are found mostly in animal fats—lard, butter and other dairy products and meat, for example—whereas monounsaturated and polyunsaturated fatty acids come mostly from vegetable sources.

Cholesterol is another member of the lipid family. It is a structural component of cell membranes. Some hormones and vitamin D can be formed from cholesterol. The body can make sufficient cholesterol to meet its needs. The main dietary sources of cholesterol are egg yolks, meat, poultry, shellfish, and whole-milk dairy products. In fact, cholesterol is found only in food of animal origin.

Since cholesterol is a fat-soluble compound, it does not float freely in the blood stream, which is mostly water. Instead, cholesterol travels through the blood stream in gigantic molecules made of fat and protein and called lipoproteins. Most of the blood cholesterol is carried in low-density lipoproteins (LDL). Cholesterol is also carried in high-density lipoproteins (HDL). Cholesterol in LDL and HDL is called, respectively, LDL-cholesterol and HDL-cholesterol. The term "total serum cholesterol" refers to the sum of cholesterol in all the lipoproteins. Medical experts strongly recommend that total serum cholesterol be below 200 milligrams per deciliter (mg/dl).

Protein is the major structural material in almost all living tissue except bones. Hair, skin, nails, and muscles are mostly protein. There are thousands of different proteins in the human body, each with a unique function, but they are all made from smaller units called **amino acids.** The body breaks down dietary protein into amino acids and then uses the amino acids in proteins. All told, there are 20 common amino acids in proteins. The body can manufacture 11 of them, but it must obtain the other 9, the so-called **essential amino acids,** from food. Animal proteins, except for gelatin, and soy proteins contain all the essential amino acids in sufficient quantities and are known as **complete proteins.** Most plant proteins are low in one or more of the essential amino acids, and so it is necessary to combine different protein sources to make up for these shortages. For example, peanut butter and bread combined are a complete protein source. So, too, are rice and beans when eaten in the same meal. Such combinations are called **complementary proteins.**

Carbohydrates are the body's best source of energy, and, in fact, they are the most important source of calories for much of the world's population because of their relatively low cost and wide availability. For our purposes, there are three types of carbohydrates: **simple carbohydrates, digestible complex carbohydrates,** and **indigestible complex carbohydrates**. Simple carbohydrates, such as glucose, fructose, sucrose, and lactose, are also called **sugars.** Some sugars taste sweet—such as those in table sugar, honey, fruits, molasses, and maple syrup, whereas others, such as those in milk and malt, have little taste at all. The body readily digests and metabolizes simple carbohydrates.

Complex carbohydrates, or **polysaccharides,** are large molecules made from hundreds of sugar molecules hooked together. In essence, sugar molecules are the building blocks of carbohydrates in the same way that amino acids are the building blocks of proteins. Starches are the most abundant polysaccharides in the diet and occur in many foods, including cereals, breads, dry beans, peas, and potatoes. The body digests polysaccharides into sugars.

Indigestible complex carbohydrates, also called **fiber** or **roughage,** are large molecules as well, but the sugar building blocks are linked together in such a way that the body cannot break them apart. Because of this, fiber does not supply energy or nutrients to the body, but it does aid in digestion and elimination. Cellulose and pectin, the two most important indigestible complex carbohydrates, are plentiful in bran, whole-grain cereals and breads, fruits, and vegetables.

Vitamins fall into two families, **fat-soluble vitamins** and **water-soluble vitamins**. Fat-soluble vitamins are often found together with fats in food. Vitamins A, D, E, and K are fat-soluble vitamins. Because water-soluble vitamins mix readily with water, excess water-soluble vitamins are not stored in the body but are washed out in urine. Vitamins C (ascorbic acid), B_1 (thiamin), B_2 (riboflavin), niacin, B_6 (pyridoxine), pantothenic acid, biotin, folacin, and B_{12} (cobalamin) are water-soluble vitamins.

Minerals, or **mineral salts,** have a variety of uses throughout the body and are involved in almost every aspect of its functioning. The minerals calcium, phosphorus, and magnesium are required in relatively large amounts. Calcium, for example, is the most abundant mineral in the body and accounts for nearly 2 percent of body weight. More than 99 percent of the body's calcium is in the bones and teeth, but calcium is also essential for nerves and muscles to work properly.

The body also requires smaller, or trace, amounts of at least 10 other minerals. These **trace elements** include chromium, cobalt, copper, fluoride, iodine, iron, manganese, molybdenum, selenium, sulfur, and zinc. All trace elements are toxic if too much is consumed over long periods of time.

Three other minerals, known as **electrolytes,** are important components of all body fluids. These minerals are sodium, potassium, and chloride. Table salt is the compound sodium chloride. Meat, peanuts, potatoes, and many fruits and vegetables are rich in potassium.

CHAPTER

3

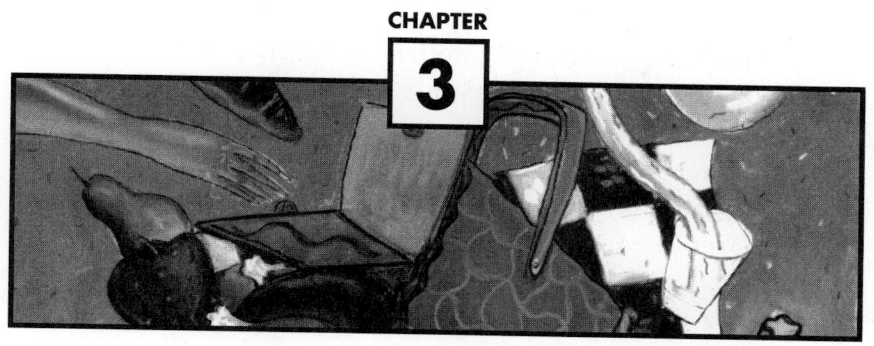

THE FOOD WE EAT

You are at the dinner table. On your plate are a roasted skinless chicken breast half topped with 1/2 cup spaghetti sauce, 1/2 cup brown rice, and a large pile (2 cups) of fresh, steamed string beans. At least that is what your eyes see and your nose smells—and your taste buds are about to experience. But just for a moment, let's look at this delicious dinner as your body sees it: a huge collection of matter to process, providing both energy and nutrients.

Food energy: 475 calories	Calcium: 174 mg
Protein: 36.4 g*	Phosphorus: 413 mg
Carbohydrate: 63 g	Sodium: 690 mg
Fat: 11 g	Potassium: 1522 mg
Saturated fat: 2.2 g	Vitamin A: 1522 I.U.†
Monounsaturated fat: 4.4 g	Vitamin C: 38 mg
Polyunsaturated fat: 3.0 g	Thiamin: 0.42 mg
Cholesterol: 73 mg	Riboflavin: 0.42 mg
Iron: 5.4 mg	Niacin: 16.5 mg

*There are approximately 28 grams (g) in 1 ounce, or approximately 0.035 ounce in 1 g; 1 mg equals one-thousandth of a gram.

†I.U. stands for international unit, a standard measurement of vitamin A content.

In addition, other vitamins and minerals are present in small amounts.

This meal is not only delicious but also nutritious, and if most of your meals were as healthful as this one you would be doing a great deal to help to reduce your risk for many chronic diseases. Fat in this meal accounts for only 21 percent of the calories, and saturated fat under 5 percent. Both of those figures are well below the guidelines in Chapter 2. The cholesterol content of the meal is low, too. In addition, there is relatively little salt in the meal, but it is high in potassium and vitamin A.

To choose healthful meals like this—and avoid the perils of a diet high in fat, cholesterol, sugar, and salt, and low in carbohydrates, potassium, and calcium—you must know something about the nutrients food contains.

WHAT'S IN FOOD?

As far as the body is concerned, food is made of various nutrients, and a large number of substances that have no nutrient value. Nutrients are the materials the body needs to build itself and stay in top working order. Some of these nutrients—primarily carbohydrates and fats, but also protein—provide energy. Others—protein and minerals—are building materials. Still others—vitamins and some trace elements and fatty acids—are necessary for the chemical reactions that produce energy to move muscles or carry out the regulation of body metabolism. To operate at its best, the body needs these nutrients in the right amounts. Too much or too little can—and often does—result in the body dysfunctioning. That's what we know as disease.

Understanding what food is made of is important if you are to provide your body with the right balance of nutrients. But you do not have to know every last detail of the nutritional composition of your food, or even the biochemical processes your body uses to convert food nutrients into energy and muscle and bones. In a way, you can treat learning how to eat better as you would approach learning to drive a car. To drive, you need to know the traffic laws and you need to know how to operate the gas pedal, brake pedal, steering wheel, and turn signals. But you do not need to understand how gasoline burns in a car's engine or how the transmission works.

So here is a brief primer on nutrition that will help you follow the guidelines in Chapter 2.

Food Energy

Just as a car needs gasoline to run, your body needs fuel to do all the things it must do every day. That fuel, of course, comes from food. The usable energy in food is measured in units called **kilocalories** or, simply, **calories.** About two-thirds of the energy the body uses goes to keeping body temperature constant, repairing internal organs and skin, keeping the heart beating and lungs breathing, and ensuring the proper chemical balance inside and outside the body's cells. Most adults need between 1300 and 1800 calories a day just to stay alive without any physical activity at all. The other third of the energy is used for moving the body through its daily activities, dressing, walking, sitting, exercising, and all the other muscle-using activities that we do.

How many additional calories we need to eat depends on what we do during the day. The number of calories your body burns to carry out an activity depends on your weight, how long you do the activity, and how much work the activity takes.

For example, washing the dishes uses about one-half calorie an hour for every pound of body weight. So when a 150-pound man washes the dishes for 15 minutes, his body burns almost 19 calories. Reading aloud to his children for half an hour requires another 15 calories. He uses about the same amount of energy every day just to eat, and the 15 minutes it takes him to get dressed in the morning and undressed at night takes an additional 11 or so calories. But riding his bicycle at a moderate pace for an hour burns about 165 calories. His wife, who weighs only 120 pounds, uses about 130 calories riding at his side.

In general, you can figure your approximate daily energy needs using one of the following equations:

For women: little physical activity: 960 + 3.8 times weight
moderate activity: 1120 + 4.5 times weight
regular exercise or manual labor: 1280 + 5.1 times weight

For men: little physical activity: 1080 + 5.5 times weight
moderate activity: 1260 + 6.4 times weight
regular exercise or manual labor: 1440 + 7.3 times weight

For example, if our 150-pound man rides his bicycle every day for an hour, his daily energy need is a little over 2500 calories a day (1440 + 7.3 times 150 = 2535). Similarly, his 120-pound wife needs almost 1900 calories a day if she exercises every day as well. If they were both couch potatoes who worked at desk jobs all day, their energy needs would drop significantly: he would need 1900 calories a day, and she would only need about 1400 calories.

Not all nutrients contain the same amount of calories (see Table 3.1). One gram of protein provides 4 calories of energy. So does 1 gram of carbohydrate. One gram of fat, however, provides 9 calories, and 1 gram of alcohol yields 7 calories.

Let's look at the practical consequences of the different calorie contents of carbohydrates, protein, and fat by comparing the calorie and nutrient content of a cup of ice cream, a cup of frozen yogurt, and a cup of ice milk (see Figure 3.1).

TABLE 3.1 Energy Yield of Fat, Protein, Carbohydrate, and Alcohol

	Calories Provided Per Gram
Fat	9
Protein	4
Carbohydrate	4
Alcohol	7

Ice cream, frozen yogurt, and ice milk are not much different in the amount of protein they contain, but the fat and carbohydrate content of the three desserts is quite different: 14 g of fat in ice cream compared with only 8 g of fat in frozen yogurt, and 7 g in ice milk. That is a difference of 6 or 7 g of fat, or about 54 to 63 calories (6 g of fat times 9 calories per gram equals 54 calories). Most foods high in calories are also high in fat.

It is not just desserts that contain a lot of fat. In the dinner at the beginning of this chapter, the food that contributed the majority of the fat was the chicken. Even so, a skinless chicken breast has only about 5.5 g of fat.

The human body uses fat as its primary means of storing energy. When the body needs to take energy out of its reserves, it preferentially uses its fat stores. It does not convert protein as a primary fuel source until most of the fat is gone. If on a given day your body needs to burn more energy than you eat, it converts some of the stored fat, at 9 calories per gram. That is why exercising regularly can help a person lose weight. On the other hand, if you eat more calories on a given day than your body uses, the body uses the surplus energy to make fat molecules and stores them in the various fatty tissues in your body. That is why you gain weight when you regularly eat more calories than your body uses.

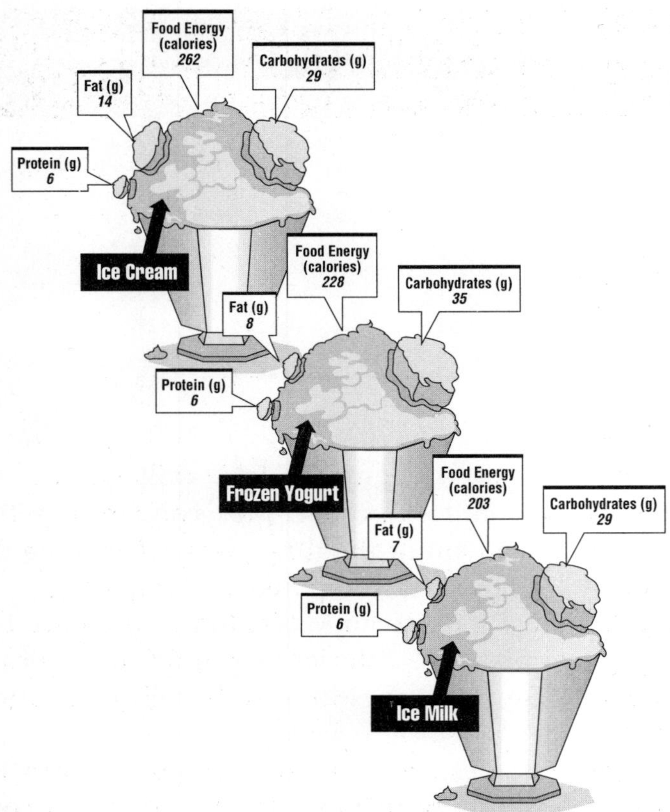

FIGURE 3.1 Comparison of calorie and nutrient content in 1 cup of ice cream, frozen yogurt, and ice milk. SOURCE: U.S. Department of Agriculture, Human Nutrition Information Service.

Carbohydrates

In the *Eat for Life* eating pattern, the most important source of food energy is **carbohydrates**. They are also the least expensive source of calories, which is why the great majority of the world's population relies on carbohydrates to meet much of their daily energy needs.

Carbohydrates are among the most plentiful substances in the world, particularly in the plant kingdom. Plants are about 10 to 15 percent carbohydrate, whereas animals, including humans, contain a mere 1 percent carbohydrate.

Carbohydrates are a family of compounds made solely of the three elements carbon, hydrogen, and oxygen. These elements are arranged into rings, and the rings can be strung together into chains that are two rings to thousands of rings long (see Figure 3.2).

Scientists distinguish carbohydrates as being either **simple carbohydrates** (sugars)—containing one or two rings (**monosaccharides** or **disaccharides**)—or **complex carbohydrates**—with many rings (**polysaccharides**). In addition, complex carbohydrates can be **digestible** (**starches**) or **indigestible** (**fiber** or **roughage**), depending on how the rings are hooked together.

Glucose, sucrose, fructose, maltose, and lactose are common sugars. The body can covert all of these sugars directly into energy, or it can use them to make fats. Glucose and fructose are made of one ring and are called monosaccharides. They are found in honey and fruit.

Sucrose, maltose, and lactose have two rings and are called disaccharides. When the body digests these sugars, it splits them into monosaccharides. Sucrose, made of one molecule of glucose hooked to one molecule of fructose, is what we call table sugar. It is found in molasses, in maple syrup, and in fruits. Maltose, consisting of two glucose molecules

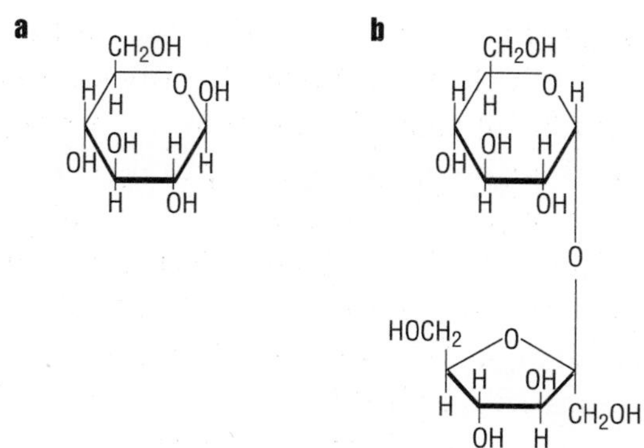

FIGURE 3.2 Structure for (a) monosaccharide glucose, and (b) disaccharide sucrose.

hooked together, is found in sprouting grains, malted milk, malted cereals, and some corn syrups. Lactose, or milk sugar, consists of one molecule of glucose and one molecule of another monosaccharide called galactose.

Sucrose and fructose are the sugars added during food processing. Corn syrups, used in many baked goods, get their sweetness from glucose and maltose. In recent years, food processors have learned how to make high-fructose corn syrups by rearranging the glucose ring to make fructose. High-fructose corn syrups have replaced much of the sucrose in most soda pops.

Starches, made of hundreds, even thousands, of glucose molecules, are the most common digestible polysaccharides in the diet. They are also the major source of energy in the human diet. Grains, beans, and some fruits and vegetables are rich sources of starch. For example, almost 90 percent of the calories in a potato and 73 percent of the calories in pinto beans come from starch.

In the digestive system, the large starch molecules are broken down, or digested, into individual glucose molecules. Glucose, not the original starch molecules, is absorbed from the digestive tract into the blood stream. When a person says he has "high blood sugar," he is talking about the amount of glucose in the blood stream, that is the blood sugar level.

Fiber is a complex mixture of many indigestible substances—most of which are nonstarch polysaccharides—that make up the structural material of plants. Among these are cellulose, hemicellulose, pectin, lignin, gums (such as guar and locust bean, common food additives used to improve the texture of some foods), and mucilage. Some processed foods contain carrageenan and alginates, indigestible polysaccharides produced by algae. Lignin is an indigestible plant product, but it is not a carbohydrate.

Pectins, gums, mucilages, and some hemicelluloses dissolve in water and are sometimes called soluble fiber. At least part of the fiber in oat and rice bran is soluble fiber. Cellulose, most hemicelluloses, and lignins do not dissolve in water and are known as insoluble fiber. Wheat bran, for example, is mostly insoluble fiber.

The main difference between indigestible polysaccharides and starch is that in both soluble and insoluble fiber the chemical links that hold the individual molecules together as a chain are resistant to the processes of the human digestive system. Thus they provide little food energy to the body. Humans cannot digest grass because it is mostly indigestible complex carbohydrate. Cows and sheep can use grass as food because their stomachs contain bacteria that digest these carbohydrates, releasing simple sugars that are absorbed into the animals' blood streams. Though fiber has little energy value for humans, it seems to be necessary for the large intestine to function at its peak.

In general, foods with a high fiber content include wholegrain breads and cereals, fruits, vegetables, beans, peas, and nuts. Fruit skins, seeds, berries, and the bran layers of cereal grains are richer sources of fiber than the rest of these foods.

Fats

In the *Eat for Life* eating pattern, **fats** take second place to carbohydrates as an energy source. Fats are a large family of compounds that are made mostly of the elements carbon and hydrogen, with a small amount of oxygen. The major fat in food is triglyceride, a molecule of glycerol with three fatty acids attached (see Figure 3.3).

Foods that are almost pure fat include cooking oil, lard, butter, margarine, and shortening. Foods that contain significant amounts of fat include meat, dairy products, chocolate, cakes, pies, cookies, nuts, and a few fruits and vegetables—coconut and avocado, for example.

One characteristic of fats is that they do not mix with or dissolve in water. Instead, fat molecules tend to cluster

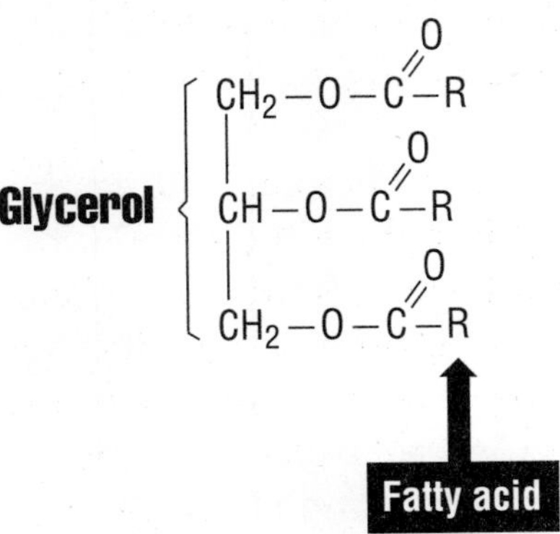

FIGURE 3.3 A triglyceride. The "R" represents fatty acids chemically bound to the glycerol backbone of the triglyceride.

together with other fat molecules. Fats are soluble in organic solvents like benzene or ether.

Fatty acids come in a variety of sizes, and all fat in foods contains a mixture of these various fatty acids. Some fatty acids contain as few as 4 carbon atoms, whereas others are made of as many as 20 or more strung together in a line. The other way in which fatty acids differ from one another is in the number of hydrogen atoms they contain per carbon atom. For example, the four fatty acids shown in Figure 3.4 all contain 16 or 18 carbon atoms and 2 oxygen atoms. Oleic, linoleic, and linolenic acids all have 18 carbons and 2 oxygens, but they have different numbers of hydrogen atoms.

Palmitic acid (Figure 3.4a) is found in meats, butter fat, shortening, and some vegetable oils. Palmitic acid is a **saturated fatty acid,** one that has the maximum number of hydrogen atoms—2—attached to every carbon atom, except for those on each end. In effect, the molecule is "saturated" with hydrogen atoms. Other saturated fatty acids found in food include stearic acid (18 carbon atoms), myristic acid (14 carbon atoms), and lauric acid (12 carbon atoms). Fats high in saturated fatty acids are usually solid at room temperature and certainly at refrigerator temperature.

In oleic acid (Figure 3.4b), there are 2 hydrogen atoms missing in the middle of the molecule, 1 from each of 2 adjoining carbon atoms. The place where this occurs is called an unsaturation. Since oleic acid has one unsaturation, it is called a **monounsaturated fatty acid.** Oleic acid is the predominant monounsaturated fatty acid in food. Olive oil, peanut oil, and canola oil are particularly good sources of oleic acid.

The last two fatty acids in Figure 3.4 are missing still more hydrogen atoms, again from adjacent pairs of carbon atoms. Since these fatty acids have more than one unsaturation, they are called **polyunsaturated fatty acids**. The polyunsaturated fatty acid with two unsaturations is called linoleic acid, and the polyunsaturated fatty acid with three unsaturations is called linolenic acid. Linoleic acid is called an essential fatty

a

```
    H   H   H   H   H   H   H   H   H   H   H   H   H   H   H
    |   |   |   |   |   |   |   |   |   |   |   |   |   |   |      O
H - C - C - C - C - C - C - C - C - C - C - C - C - C - C - C - C //
    |   |   |   |   |   |   |   |   |   |   |   |   |   |   |      \ OH
    H   H   H   H   H   H   H   H   H   H   H   H   H   H   H
```

b

```
    H   H   H   H   H   H   H   H   H   H   H   H   H   H   H   H   H
    |   |   |   |   |   |   |   |   |   |   |   |   |   |   |   |   |      O
H - C - C - C - C - C - C - C - C - C = C - C - C - C - C - C - C - C - C //
    |   |   |   |   |   |   |   |           |   |   |   |   |   |   |      \ OH
    H   H   H   H   H   H   H   H           H   H   H   H   H   H   H
```

c

```
    H   H   H   H   H   H   H   H   H   H   H   H   H   H   H   H   H
    |   |   |   |   |   |   |   |   |   |   |   |   |   |   |   |   |      O
H - C - C - C - C - C - C = C - C - C = C - C - C - C - C - C - C - C - C //
    |   |   |   |   |           |           |   |   |   |   |   |   |      \ OH
    H   H   H   H   H           H           H   H   H   H   H   H   H
```

d

```
    H   H   H   H   H   H   H   H   H   H   H   H   H   H   H   H   H
    |   |   |   |   |   |   |   |   |   |   |   |   |   |   |   |   |      O
H - C - C - C = C - C - C = C - C - C = C - C - C - C - C - C - C - C - C //
    |   |           |           |           |   |   |   |   |   |   |      \ OH
    H   H           H           H           H   H   H   H   H   H   H
```

FIGURE 3.4 Comparison of the structure of four fatty acids: (a) palmitic, (b) oleic, (c) linoleic, and (d) linolenic acids.

acid because the body cannot make it and must meet its need for it from food sources. Scientists believe that linolenic acid may prove to be an essential nutrient as well.

Foods from the plant kingdom, with the notable exceptions of palm oil and coconut, are good sources of polyunsaturated fatty acids. Seafood is rich in monounsaturated fatty acids and polyunsaturated fatty acids. Fats with a large percentage of monounsaturated fatty acids and polyunsaturated fatty acids are usually liquid even when refrigerated.

Polyunsaturated fatty acids are further classified by where the unsaturations exist in the fatty acid molecule. You may have heard of omega-3 fatty acids, the main polyunsaturated fatty acid in many fish oils. All this term means is that the first unsaturation occurs at the third carbon atom from the omega end of the fatty acid, the end with 3 hydrogen atoms. Eicosapentaenoic acid (shown in Figure 3.5) is one of the chief omega-3 fatty acids in fish oil. If you count the carbon atoms starting at the omega end, you can see why linoleic acid is called an omega-6 fatty acid.

If you read food labels, you have probably seen the term "partially hydrogenated vegetable oil." This means that hydrogen atoms have been added to unsaturated fatty acids by means of a chemical process known as hydrogenation. This reaction eliminates some of the unsaturations; monounsaturated fatty acids become saturated fatty acids, and polyunsaturated fatty acids become monounsaturated fatty acids and saturated fatty acids. Vegetable oils are partially hydrogenated to make them solid at room temperature. Vegetable shortening and margarine are two examples of partially hydrogenated vegetable oils.

Unsaturated fatty acids in foods exist chiefly in the *cis* configuration, in which the hydrogen atoms are on the same side of the double bond. When fats and oils are partially hydrogenated during commercial processing, varying amounts of the *trans* configuration form. In the *trans* configuration, the hydrogen atoms are on opposite sides of the double bond.

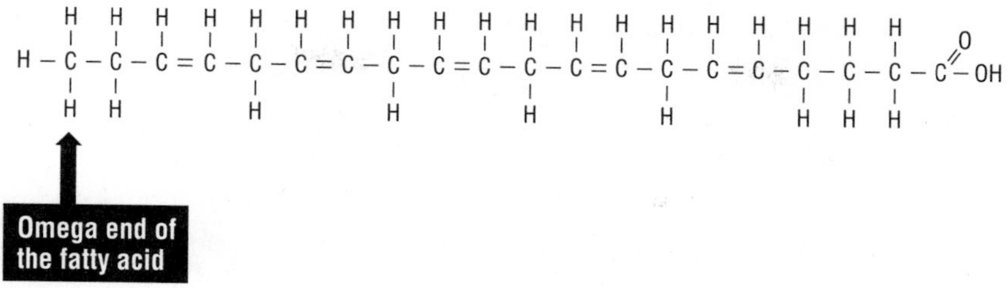

```
    H   H   H   H   H   H   H   H   H   H   H   H   H   H   H   H   H   H   H
    |   |   |   |   |   |   |   |   |   |   |   |   |   |   |   |   |   |   |   O
H - C - C - C = C - C - C = C - C - C = C - C - C = C - C - C = C - C - C - C - C//
    |   |           |           |           |           |           |   |   |    \OH
    H   H           H           H           H           H           H   H   H
```

Omega end of the fatty acid

FIGURE 3.5 An omega-3 fatty acid: eicosapentaenoic acid.

Although small amounts of *trans* fatty acids occur naturally in milk and butter, the large increase in the use of partially hydrogenated vegetable oils has resulted in increases in *trans* fatty acids in foods. As yet, there are no reliable data on the *trans* fatty acid intake by the U.S. population, and estimates vary from 7 to 12 g per person per day.

Remember that all fats contain a mixture of fatty acids. Some have more of one kind of fatty acid than another kind. Beef fat, for example, contains more saturated fatty acids than monounsaturated or polyunsaturated fatty acids. Olive oil contains both saturated fatty acids and polyunsaturated fatty acids, but over half its fatty acids are monounsaturated, and most of that is oleic acid.

Cholesterol

There are a number of substances in food that are not exactly fats but, like fats, do not mix with water. One of these substances is **cholesterol** (see Figure 3.6).

Cholesterol exists in foods of animal origin and in the body, where it is an important component of many tissues, particularly the brain and nervous system. Cholesterol is found in all body cells as part of the structure of cell membranes. The body also uses cholesterol to make bile acids, various hormones, and vitamin D. Cholesterol is not an essential nutrient, however, because the body can manufacture all it needs.

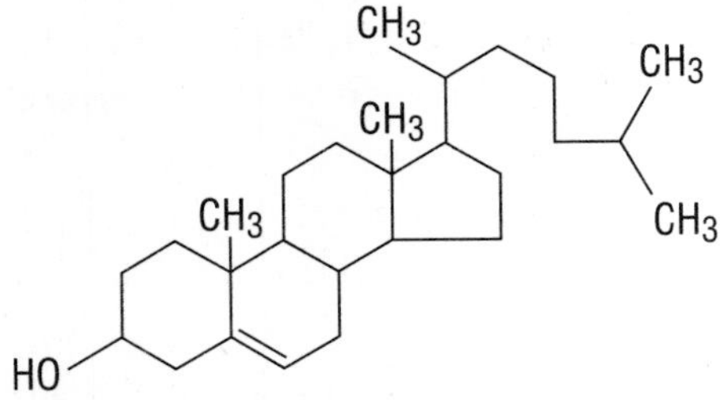

FIGURE 3.6 Cholesterol.

Nevertheless, the U.S. diet has many sources of cholesterol, including egg yolks, liver, meat, certain shellfish, and whole-milk dairy products. Cholesterol is not found in plant foods.

Because cholesterol does not dissolve in water, it moves through the blood stream in clusters of molecules made of fat and protein called **lipoproteins**. Most of the cholesterol in the body is carried by three types of lipoproteins: **high-density lipoprotein (HDL)**, **low-density lipoprotein (LDL)**, and **very-low-density lipoprotein (VLDL)**. Cholesterol found in HDL is called **HDL-cholesterol**, and cholesterol found in LDL is called **LDL-cholesterol**. The term **total serum cholesterol** refers to the sum of HDL-, LDL-, and VLDL-cholesterol in the blood stream. Medical experts consider a total serum cholesterol level below 200 milligrams per deciliter (mg/dl) to be desirable.

Protein

If carbohydrates and fat are the body's energy sources, then **proteins** are the body's building blocks. If you do not count water, protein accounts for about three-quarters of the weight in most human tissues. Hair, skin, nails, and muscle are mostly protein, and bone contains a significant amount of protein as well. Certain proteins, called **enzymes**, perform the countless chemical reactions needed to produce energy to keep your body operating and to produce the thousands of different molecules that are present in muscle, bone, skin, hair, and organs.

Protein is composed of smaller chemical units called **amino acids**. Amino acids are made of the elements carbon, hydrogen, oxygen, nitrogen, and sometimes sulfur. There are 20 different amino acids that when hooked together in various numbers and combinations make up the thousands of different proteins in the human body. The body can make enough of all but 9 of these, the so-called **essential amino acids**.

In practice, protein is the only source of the essential amino acids in the diet. When you eat a piece of chicken, your digestive system breaks the protein molecules in that chunk of chicken muscle into individual amino acids. These are absorbed into the blood stream and transported to all the cells in the body. Enzymes and other biological molecules inside a cell reassemble the amino acids into those proteins that the cell needs.

The body does not store significant amounts of amino acids, and so we have to eat protein regularly. Meat is a rich source of protein, since muscle is protein with fat mixed in. So, too, are dairy products. Beans, nuts, and cereal grains are also good sources of protein. Worldwide, people get most of their protein from vegetable sources, rather than the animal sources that provide most of the protein in U.S. diets.

Vitamins

Vitamins are a group of diverse compounds that the body needs in small amounts to remain healthy. They are used in a variety of biochemical processes. Vitamin K, for example, plays an important role in blood clotting, and vitamin D is involved in absorbing calcium and thus maintaining the bones in good condition. Some of the functions of the vitamins are listed together with food sources in Table 3.2.

When they were first discovered around the turn of the century, vitamins were classified according to whether or not they dissolved in water. The **fat-soluble vitamins** are vitamins A, D, E, and K. The **water-soluble vitamins** are vitamin

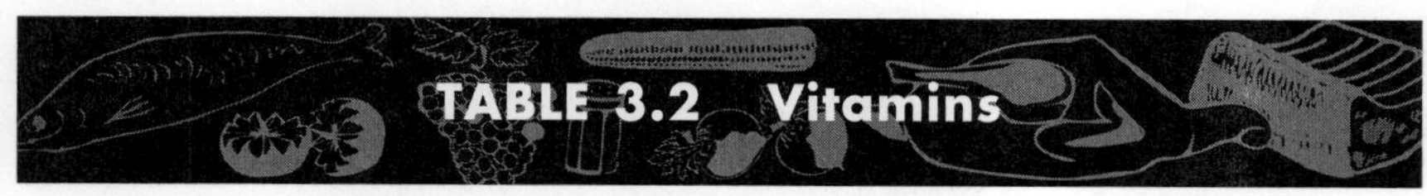

TABLE 3.2 Vitamins

Vitamin	Functions	Food Sources
Fat-Soluble Vitamins		
Vitamin A	Maintains normal vision and healthy skin and mucous membranes; necessary for normal growth and for reproduction	Liver, butter, whole milk, egg yolks; margarine, skim milk, and certain breakfast cereals are fortified with vitamin A; the body also makes vitamin A from carotenoids, compounds present in dark-green leafy vegetables, yellow and orange vegetables, and fruit
Vitamin D	Promotes calcium and phosphorus absorption from the intestines; influences bone growth	Liver, butter, fatty fish, egg yolks; milk is fortified with vitamin D
Vitamin E	Antioxidant that prevents cells from being damaged by various biochemical reactions that occur naturally	Best sources are vegetable oils; also found in nuts, seeds, whole grains, and wheat germ
Vitamin K	Aids in blood clotting	Best source is dark-green leafy vegetables; also found in cereals, dairy products, meat, and fruits
Water-Soluble Vitamins		
Vitamin C	Promotes growth of connective tissues; antioxidant	Citrus fruits, tomatoes, broccoli, green peppers, strawberries, melons, cabbage, and leafy green vegetables; vitamin C is destroyed when foods are overcooked or cooked in large amounts of water
Thiamin (Vitamin B_1)	Aids in obtaining energy from carbohydrates	Meat, eggs, beans, and whole grains; enriched breads and cereals

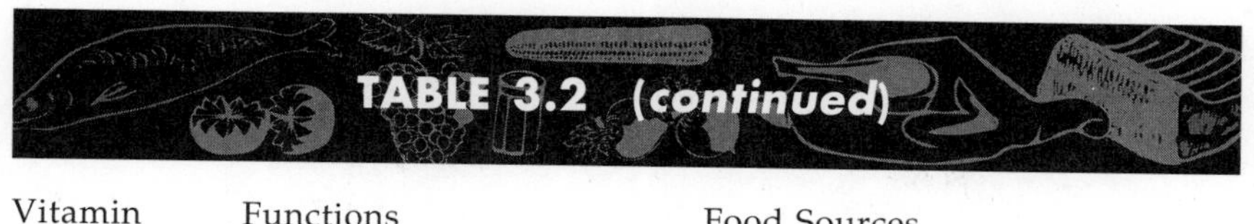

Vitamin	Functions	Food Sources
Riboflavin (Vitamin B_2)	Aids in energy production and in many other biochemical processes	Liver, milk, and dark-green leafy vegetables; whole grains and enriched breads and cereals
Niacin	Aids in energy production from fats, proteins, and carbohydrates; aids in manufacture of fatty acids	Grain products, meat, poultry, fish, nuts, and beans
Pyridoxine (Vitamin B_6)	Aids in manufacture of amino acids; aids in energy production from protein	Meat, poultry, fish, grain products, and fruits and vegetables
Cobalamin (Vitamin B_{12})	Aids in DNA synthesis, and in energy production from fatty acids and carbohydrates; aids in production of amino acids	Meat, milk and milk products, and eggs
Folacin	Aids in manufacture of genetic material in cells; aids in production of amino acids	Dark-green leafy vegetables, liver, and fruits
Biotin	Aids in energy production	Egg yolks, liver, beans, and nuts
Pantothenic acid	Aids in energy production; aids in the manufacture of fatty acids; participates in a wide variety of other biochemical processes	Most foods

C and the eight B vitamins—thiamin, riboflavin, niacin, pyridoxine, pantothenic acid, biotin, folacin, and cobalamin.

Fat-soluble vitamins are found in association with fats in foods, and they are also absorbed out of the digestive system along with fats. The body can store variable amounts of the fat-soluble vitamins. It is possible to consume too much of some fat-soluble vitamins so that they build up in the body to toxic levels. Vitamin A and vitamin D poisonings are not unknown and can cause serious illness, and even death.

Some vitamins are manufactured in the body. Vitamin D is made in the skin when exposed to sunlight. Bacteria that live in the human intestine produce vitamin K, which is then absorbed into the blood stream.

With the notable exception of vitamin B_{12}, the body stores little of the water-soluble vitamins, and so you must get these substances in your diet regularly. Taking large amounts of these vitamins is futile, however, because the excess is carried in the blood stream to the kidneys and excreted in the urine.

Minerals

Like vitamins, minerals play a variety of roles in the body. Some minerals, such as calcium and phosphorus, are present in the body in relatively large amounts and are sometimes called **macrominerals.** Other minerals, such as iron and copper, are needed in much lower amounts and are called **trace elements.** Three macrominerals—sodium, potassium, and chloride—are sometimes called **electrolytes,** because they help maintain the proper electrical balance in cells and body fluids. Some of the functions of minerals are listed together with food sources in Table 3.3.

Whereas all the other nutrients discussed so far are relatively big molecules, minerals are simple chemicals made of single atoms or **salts** made up of a few atoms. Together, minerals account for only about 4 percent of body weight.

Salts are associations of positive and negative components called ions. Table salt, for example, is made from positively charged sodium ions and negatively charged chloride ions—the chemical name for table salt is sodium chloride. When

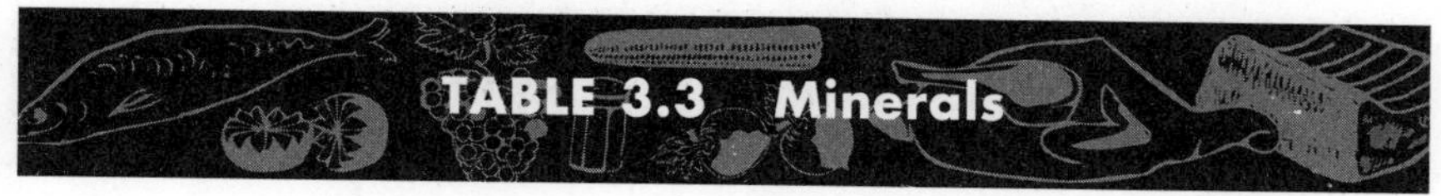

Mineral	Functions	Food Sources
Calcium	The most abundant mineral in the body, 99 percent is in bones; is also important in muscle function	Dairy products, bones of sardines and canned salmon, dark-green leafy vegetables, and lime-processed tortillas
Chloride	Is a component of stomach acid; aids in maintaining fluid balance in cells	Table salt, eggs, meat, and milk
Chromium	Works with insulin to promote carbohydrate and fat metabolism	Liver and other organ meats, brewer's yeast, whole grains, and nuts
Copper	Aids in energy production; aids in absorption of iron from digestive tract; forms dark pigment in hair and skin	Liver, meat, whole grains, and nuts
Fluoride	Strengthens teeth and bones	Some natural waters, fluoridated water, and tea
Iodine	Is part of the thyroid hormones that regulate metabolism	Iodized table salt, ocean seafood, dairy products, and commercially made bread
Iron	Aids in energy production; helps to carry oxygen in the blood stream and muscles	Meat, poultry, fish, nuts, whole and enriched grain products, and green vegetables
Magnesium	Is necessary for nerve function, bone formation, and general metabolic processes	Grain products, vegetables, dairy products, fish, meat, and poultry
Manganese	Aids in regulation of carbohydrate metabolism and in general metabolic processes	Cereals and most other plant foods

continued

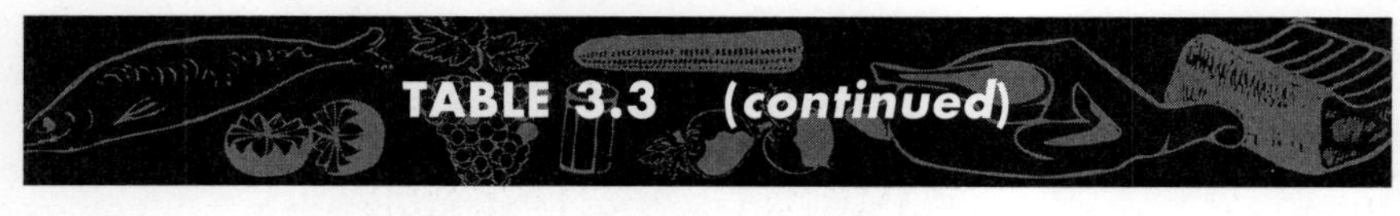

TABLE 3.3 (*continued*)

Mineral	Functions	Food Sources
Molybdenum	Aids in energy production	Meat, beans, and cereals
Phosphorus	Aids in bone formation, general metabolic processes, and energy production and storage	Dairy products, meat, poultry, fish, and grain products
Potassium	Is necessary to maintain fluid balance in cells, transmit nerve signals, and produce energy	Fruits and vegetables, nuts, grains, and seeds
Selenium	Protects cells against harmful reactions involving oxygen; aids in detoxifying toxic substances	Meat, ocean fish, and wheat
Sodium	Is necessary to maintain fluid balance in cells, transmit nerve signals, and relax muscles	Table salt and salt added to food during processing
Zinc	Is necessary for cell reproduction and tissue repair and growth	Oysters and other shellfish, meat, poultry, eggs, hard cheeses, milk, yogurt, beans, nuts, and whole-grain cereals

table salt is dissolved in water, it separates into sodium and chloride ions again. Sodium bicarbonate is the salt we call baking soda. In this book the term "salt" will refer only to the compound sodium chloride. All other salts will be referred to by their chemical names.

HOW DIET HAS CHANGED OVER TIME

For most of human history, the quest for sufficient food was the chief occupation of the earth's people. Our early ancestors were hunter-gatherers, searching for edible plants and killing the occasional animal. Archeologists have found evidence suggesting that the early human diet was about 35 percent meat and 65 percent plant food, though little of it was cereal grains. These people ate very little fat—they ate no dairy products and the meat they ate contained only about 4 percent fat—and only low levels of sodium, but their diets were rich in dietary fiber, calcium, and vitamin C.

Two things happened to change the human diet. The first took place around 10,000 B.C., when some people became farmers. For the first time, dairy products and cereal grains became a part of the diet, and the supply of meat became more predictable.

The second important change accompanied the Industrial Revolution of the late eighteenth century. The rise of factories gave birth to a new middle class of merchants and managers who had the money to afford a variety of foods. This demand prompted farmers to improve their methods and grow a wider variety of crops. The result was that the amount of food available to all people, both middle class and poor, increased. At the same time, the cost of food dropped significantly.

In the two centuries that have passed since then, the U.S. diet has undergone remarkable changes. In 1800, 95 percent of all Americans ate food that was straight off the farm, or fresh from the sea, with little processing done to it. Today, 95 percent of all Americans depend on others to produce, process, and distribute food to supermarkets. What we can eat depends mostly on what we can afford to buy.

Today, refrigerated railcars, trucks, and cargo planes make seasonal foods available year-round. A cornucopia of canned, frozen, fermented, and dried foods appears on grocery store shelves, as do the foods seen nowhere in nature that come out of our country's food laboratories, such as "fruit" drinks that have no fruit juice and "meats" made from soybeans or wheat gluten. Supermarkets now carry as many as 30,000 different items, making the U.S. diet the most varied in the world.

Given the changes that have occurred in the U.S. food supply during this century, it is surprising that Americans today have available about the same level of calories as our grandparents did at the turn of the century. At the same time, we weigh more than our grandparents, suggesting that we do not get as much exercise as was once common.

The source of the calories in the food supply has changed. Fats now provide about 40 percent of the calories in the U.S. diet, compared with only 32 percent in 1909 (see Figure 3.7). The amount of polyunsaturated fatty acids and monounsaturated

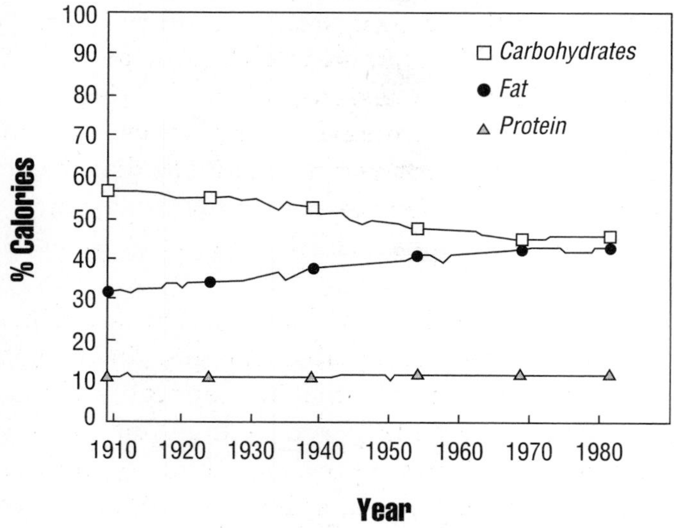

FIGURE 3.7 Percent of calories from carbohydrate, fat, and protein in the U.S. food supply since 1909. SOURCE: U.S. Department of Health and Human Services and U.S. Department of Agriculture. 1986. *Nutrition Monitoring in the United States.* U.S. Government Printing Office, Washington, D.C.

fatty acids in the U.S. diet increased more than the amount of saturated fatty acids during that period. Americans today eat about 385 mg of cholesterol a day, which is probably less than our grandparents ate because we consume fewer eggs and less butter than they did.

We also eat proportionately fewer carbohydrates than Americans did at the turn of the century; carbohydrates today account for 43 percent of the calories in the food supply, compared with 57 percent in 1909. In 1909, two-thirds of the carbohydrates in the food supply were complex polysaccharides, and one-third were simple sugars. Today, over half the carbohydrate calories are from sugars, with less than half coming from starches.

Calories from protein have remained fairly constant during this century, at about 17 percent of total calories.

What foods provide the calories in the U.S. diet? The largest share of calories comes from grain products and from meat, poultry, and fish. Fats, sweets, and beverages combined contribute about as many calories as fruit and vegetables or dairy products. Eggs, beans, nuts, and seeds combined account for the smallest proportion of calories in the U.S. diet.

Americans have also changed their eating patterns over the years. Whereas breakfast used to be the most important meal of the day, today only 53 percent of adults—and only 85 percent of children age five or younger—eat breakfast. In addition, eating out has become more common. One survey found that over half the women questioned ate out on a given day, and 88 percent ate out at least once over a 4-day period. Snacks now provide about 18 percent of the calories in the average U.S. diet.

It is commonly thought that the U.S. diet has become healthier since the last century. We live longer, grow taller, and enjoy better health than our ancestors. Diet has had some part in the health benefits we have realized over the years. Deficiency diseases are rarely seen in the United States today. But we now live longer primarily because of improved sanitation, antibiotics, and vaccinations—infectious diseases are no longer the major killers they once were. Many diseases linked in some way to diet—heart disease, high blood pressure, cancer, diabetes, dental cavities, and others—still plague us.

CHAPTER

4

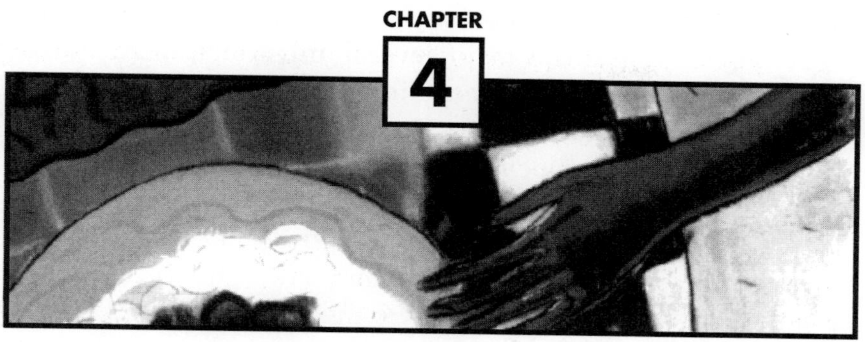

DIET AND CHRONIC DISEASE IN THE UNITED STATES

Humans have recognized that there is a connection between diet and health for centuries. As far back as 400 B.C., Hippocrates wrote about the relationship of diet to health: "The power of nutriment reaches to bone and to all parts of bone, to sinew, to vein, to artery, to muscle, to membrane, to flesh, fat, blood, phlegm, marrow, brain, spinal marrow, the intestines and all their parts. It reaches to heat, breath, and moisture."

In 1796 the British Navy instituted what was perhaps the first dietary cure for a human disease: sailors were given lime juice while at sea to cure scurvy. At the time, no one knew about vitamin C or the body's need for it, but people had made the observation that citrus fruits could prevent this life-threatening disease. But only in the past hundred years or so have we come to accept the modern concept of nutrition—that human life depends on a steady intake of a variety of specific dietary components in defined amounts. And it was not until 1932 that scientists finally isolated vitamin C from lemon juice.

Scurvy was only one of several nutritional diseases that affected many people in the United States. Others included anemia (iron deficiency), goiter (iodine deficiency), rickets (vitamin D deficiency), and pellagra (niacin deficiency). For the most part, these diseases were eradicated in the United States in the first half of this century. The introduction of "iodized" salt, for example, virtually eliminated goiter, and milk fortified with vitamin D did a great deal to solve the problem of rickets.

Today, the diet-related diseases we face are very different. They develop over a much longer time than the vitamin deficiencies of earlier times. The insidious nature of these chronic, or slow-to-develop, diseases is what makes it all the more important to pay attention to what you eat now.

How important is it for us as a nation—and you as an individual—to change our eating habits? Of the 10 leading killer diseases in the United States, 6 are connected in some way to what we eat or drink. Combined, these 6—heart disease, cancer, stroke, diabetes mellitus, chronic liver disease and cirrhosis, and atherosclerosis—accounted for nearly 1.5 million deaths in 1987, nearly 70 percent of all deaths in the United States that year (see Figure 4.1). Alcohol ingestion plays a role in two leading causes of death—accidents and suicide. Only two of the leading causes of death are not connected to what we eat or drink—chronic obstructive lung disease, and pneumonia and influenza.

This is not to say that bad eating habits alone caused 1.5 million deaths in 1987, for diet is not the only factor that causes these diseases to develop. But changing our diet for the better could go a long way to reducing the disease toll significantly.

Improving the nation's diet could also do a great deal to reduce the number of people suffering from illnesses that are serious but not immediately life-threatening. High blood pressure, obesity, dental diseases, osteoporosis, and gallstones

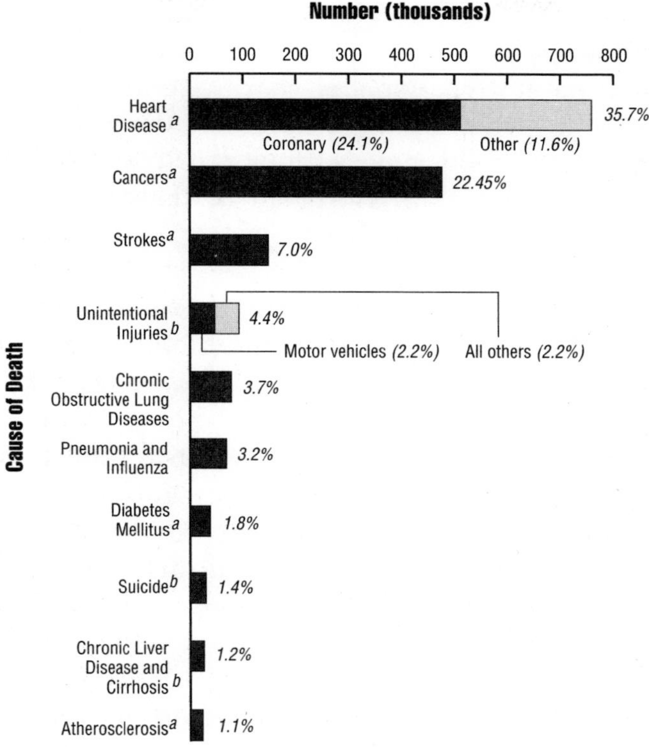

FIGURE 4.1 Estimated deaths and percent of total deaths for the 10 leading causes of death in the United States, 1987. SOURCE: U.S. Department of Health and Human Services. 1988. *The Surgeon General's Report on Nutrition and Health*. U.S. Government Printing Office, Washington, D.C.

[a]indicates causes of death in which diet plays a part.

[b]indicates causes of death in which excessive alcohol consumption plays a part.

fall into this category of diet-related chronic diseases. Over 57 million people in the United States have high blood pressure. Obesity affects 34 million people, osteoporosis 15 to 20 million. Nearly one-half million people were operated on in 1987 because of gallstones. And dental disorders, while rarely fatal, added over $21 billion to the nation's medical bill in that year. In addition, over 60 million Americans have high blood cholesterol levels, a risk factor for heart disease.

This chapter will explain what these diseases are, who gets them, and—when known—how they develop. The next five chapters will show how various nutritional factors play important roles in the development of these major chronic diseases.

ATHEROSCLEROSIS (HARDENING OF THE ARTERIES)

The number one killer in the United States is heart disease, and the number one cause of heart disease is atherosclerosis, or "hardening of the arteries." Atherosclerosis also contributes to a majority of strokes, the third leading cause of death. Therefore let's begin our discussion by examining how arteries become clogged.

Atherosclerosis is a condition of adulthood, but it starts when we are children. Lipids, particularly cholesterol and cholesterol linked to fatty acids, begin building up in the muscular walls of the arteries that carry blood throughout the body. The places where lipids accumulate are called fatty streaks.

In adolescence, fatty streaks can grow as more and more cholesterol is incorporated into the arterial walls. The body responds to the presence of fatty streaks by covering them with hard, stiff fibrous tissue and muscle, forming what are called fibrous plaques.

As we move into middle age, the fibrous plaques can continue to grow, accumulating cholesterol, fibrous tissue, and muscle cells. At some point, plaques can begin to calcify—calcium deposits form, and the plaques harden. The arteries begin to narrow, and blood has a harder time flowing through them.

At this stage, several things can happen. The worst (and a relatively common) case is when a stiff, brittle plaque cracks, causing a blood clot to form over the already obstructing deposit. Often, the additional bulk of the blood clot is enough to block the artery, which prevents blood—and the oxygen and nutrients it carries—from reaching tissues downstream from the obstruction. The tissues downstream will then die.

Fortunately, there are indications that the plaque-forming process can be prevented through dietary changes. The continued incorporation of cholesterol into the vessel walls can be arrested and may occasionally even be reversed. When that happens, plaques can actually shrink.

The key to atherosclerosis and its reversal lies with the two major carriers of cholesterol—low-density lipoprotein (LDL) and high-density lipoprotein (HDL). LDL particles carry about 60 to 70 percent of the cholesterol circulating through the blood stream, and HDL particles hold between 20 and 30 percent of the total serum cholesterol.

It turns out that LDL-cholesterol and HDL-cholesterol have quite different roles in the body. LDL-cholesterol delivers cholesterol from the liver to the millions of cells in the body. HDL-cholesterol can help to remove cholesterol from the millions of cells in the body and return it to the liver.

In the simplest terms, too much LDL-cholesterol causes cholesterol to accumulate on the walls of blood vessels, leading to fatty streaks, plaques, and blocked arteries. In societies in which the population is at a high risk of developing atherosclerosis—such as affluent Western societies—most people have relatively elevated LDL and total cholesterol levels. In addition, the level of HDL-cholesterol is an important factor in individual risk. Lowering the amount of LDL-cholesterol in the blood, and raising the level of HDL-cholesterol, can help to remove cholesterol from plaques and fatty streaks, preventing further narrowing of arteries. As is shown in Chapter 6, the levels of both LDL-cholesterol and HDL-cholesterol in the blood are important factors in whether you are at risk for heart disease, peripheral artery disease, and stroke.

HEART DISEASE

When atherosclerosis occurs in the arteries that supply blood to the heart muscle itself (the coronary arteries), the result is often coronary heart disease. Like other organs, the heart muscle needs an adequate supply of blood. If that supply is partially blocked by arterial plaque, the heart muscle does not get enough oxygen, and chest pain (called angina pectoris) can occur.

In this case, open but narrowed arteries may not be able to deliver the additional oxygen that the heart muscle requires at times of emotional excitement or physical exertion. Climbing stairs, for example, can trigger an angina attack; the pain is no different than that produced by any other muscle when it is taxed beyond its capacity.

The heart can compensate for atherosclerosis to a degree by rerouting blood from other coronary vessels, but if atherosclerosis continues unchecked even this will not keep the heart healthy. When a coronary artery becomes blocked, usually when a clot forms at a plaque deposit, the tissues downstream from the obstruction die, and this is called a myocardial infarction, or a heart attack.

About one-third of all people who suffer a heart attack die suddenly because the heart simply stops beating with any regularity. In many instances, prompt medical treatment can restore the heart's rhythm enough to keep the heart attack victim alive. Other people have a nonfatal heart attack in which the heart is damaged but does not stop beating. Within the first few hours after the heart attack, the affected part of the heart dies, and the body begins replacing the dead muscle with connective tissue. Other parts of the heart, if their blood supply is not restricted, eventually grow larger to compensate for the missing muscle.

Approximately 6.7 million people in the United States have coronary heart disease, and in 1987 over 500,000 people died from a heart attack, making it the leading cause of death.

In addition, another 725,000 people suffered a heart attack and survived. Men are more likely than women to develop coronary heart disease and suffer a fatal heart attack at a younger age, but the risk rises rapidly for women after menopause. Women get coronary heart disease about 10 years later than men, but, overall, as many women as men die from coronary heart disease in the United States. The risk of death from heart disease is greater for white men than for black men, but higher for black women than for white women.

The situation is improving, however, and the number of deaths has dropped from its high in 1967. This is true among all U.S. population groups. At least part of the reduced death toll from heart disease—some health experts estimate as much as 30 percent—can be tied to better eating habits among the U.S. public. The death rate from heart disease has also dropped, thanks in part to improved medical treatment and because fewer people are smoking cigarettes.

PERIPHERAL ARTERY DISEASE

Muscle damage from atherosclerosis can also happen in the chest, abdomen, legs, and feet, a disorder known as peripheral artery disease. If the blood supply to the legs or feet is restricted, the result is muscle tiredness, and pain upon exertion. When the blood supply to the legs and feet is completely blocked, tissue dies and gangrene results. In the chest and abdominal areas, atherosclerosis can cause the aorta—the main artery—to balloon and rupture, producing life-threatening internal bleeding.

In 1987, slightly more than 23,000 people died from peripheral artery disease, making it the tenth leading cause of death. But since peripheral artery disease is not usually a direct cause of death—it more often leads to other disorders such as aneurysms that can be fatal—health officials believe it is a larger health problem than the death toll suggests.

STROKE

When atherosclerosis affects the arteries supplying blood to the brain, a stroke can result. One type of stroke, called a cerebral thrombosis, occurs when a blood clot forms on top of an arterial plaque in a blood vessel in the neck or head. This shuts off or seriously restricts the blood supply to a part of the brain, killing the tissue there in a matter of minutes. This type of stroke typically causes paralysis on one side of the body or disturbances of speech, vision, hearing, or memory.

The exact signs and symptoms of the stroke depend on the specific parts of the brain that are affected. With physical therapy, another part of the brain can sometimes be trained to take over the task once controlled by the damaged area, restoring most or all of the lost functions. A cerebral thrombosis can be fatal, however, if the damage occurs in an area of the brain responsible for breathing.

Atherosclerosis can also cause a second type of stroke—a cerebral hemorrhage—if a plaque-covered artery becomes weak enough to rupture. This happens more frequently in people with high blood pressure, and large parts of the brain can die if the bleeding is severe enough. Cerebral hemorrhage strokes have many of the same symptoms as strokes caused by blood clots, but cerebral hemorrhages are more likely to be fatal.

About 2.7 million people in the United States have atherosclerosis of brain arteries, and in 1987 nearly 150,000 people died from a stroke, making it the third leading cause of death. Another 350,000 survive a stroke each year, and all told there are about 2 million stroke survivors in the United States. The risk of death from stroke is twice as great in blacks as whites. Even more than heart attacks, the number of deaths from stroke has declined greatly in the last 20 years, mainly due to effective control of hypertension.

HIGH BLOOD PRESSURE (HYPERTENSION)

Hardening of the brain arteries is one ingredient in the recipe for stroke. The second major element is high blood pressure, also known as hypertension. High blood pressure damages the heart, kidneys, and nervous system and increases the risk for heart attack, stroke, peripheral artery disease, and kidney disease.

Blood pressure is the force of blood against the walls of arteries. This pressure is created by the heart as it pumps blood through the body. The smaller arteries of the circulatory system are responsible for controlling blood pressure. When they contract, blood cannot pass easily through them, and so the heart must pump harder to push the blood through. This increased push increases the blood pressure in the arteries. If the blood pressure increases above normal and remains elevated, the result is high blood pressure.

In most cases, high blood pressure is apparently caused by the interaction between genetic susceptibility and lifestyle influences including high-salt diets, alcohol, and obesity. In a few cases, high blood pressure is a symptom of an underlying problem, such as kidney disease.

Whatever the cause, high blood pressure is bad because it adds to the workload of the heart and damages the lining of arteries. When the heart is forced to work harder than normal for a long period of time, it tends to become bigger. A slightly enlarged heart may function just fine, but a heart that is much larger than normal has a difficult time keeping up with the demands placed on it.

Arteries also show the wear and tear of high blood pressure. Eventually, damage to the arterial wall may contribute to the formation of arterial plaques. Eventually, the increased pressure on plaques already formed can cause them to rupture as well.

There are few apparent symptoms of high blood pressure, but it is easy to detect with a familiar device called a sphygmomanometer, or blood pressure cuff. The cuff is wrapped around the upper arm and inflated with air. This causes the cuff to squeeze against and compress a large artery in the arm, momentarily stopping the blood flow.

As the air is released from the cuff, the pressure drops to the point when blood begins to flow, the doctor or nurse listens with a stethoscope to the sound of the blood pushing through the artery. While listening and watching a gauge, two measurements are recorded: the pressure when the blood flow first is heard in the artery—the systolic pressure—and the pressure when the flow of blood becomes continuous between heartbeats—the diastolic pressure.

Both numbers, the systolic and diastolic pressures, make up a blood pressure measurement—110/70, for example. The more difficult it is for the blood to flow, the higher the numbers. Two or more readings greater than 140/90 are considered to indicate the presence of high blood pressure.

Blood pressure varies to a certain extent from day to day, and, in fact, the anxiety of being in a doctor's office can raise blood pressure. Thus doctors measure a patient's blood pressure on at least two occasions before making a diagnosis of high blood pressure. Though most cases of high blood pressure affect the diastolic pressure, some show a diastolic pressure below 90 but elevated systolic pressure. Criteria for diagnosing both cases are shown in Figure 4.2.

As many as 58 million people in the United States are thought to have high blood pressure. Some are taking medication to control high blood pressure, and others are not yet diagnosed. High blood pressure is more common among black adults than white adults and is especially high in black women.

Because of widespread publicity about the dangers of high blood pressure, the number of undiagnosed cases has dropped in the past quarter of a century, and more and more people are controlling their high blood pressure successfully. Medical experts estimate that if all cases of high blood pres-

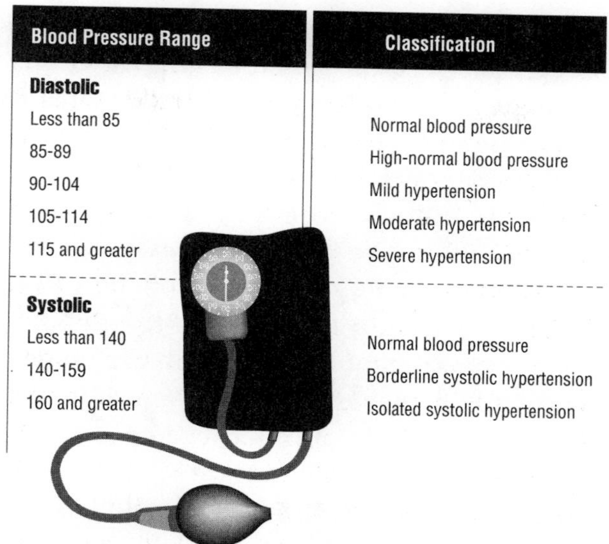

Blood Pressure Range	Classification
Diastolic	
Less than 85	Normal blood pressure
85-89	High-normal blood pressure
90-104	Mild hypertension
105-114	Moderate hypertension
115 and greater	Severe hypertension
Systolic	
Less than 140	Normal blood pressure
140-159	Borderline systolic hypertension
160 and greater	Isolated systolic hypertension

FIGURE 4.2 Criteria used to diagnose high blood pressure. SOURCE: U.S. Department of Health and Human Services. 1988. *The Surgeon General's Report on Nutrition and Health*. U.S. Government Printing Office, Washington, D.C.

sure in this country were brought under control, there would be a 20 percent drop in the total number of deaths among whites, a 30 percent drop among black men, and a 45 percent decline among black women.

CANCER

In 1987, more than 480,000 people in the United States died from cancer, making this most feared disease the number two killer. In addition, almost a million new cases of cancer were diagnosed that year. Cancer rates tend to be higher in the northeast United States and lower in rural areas, except for stomach cancer, where the reverse is true. Some cancers are more common in women, others in men.

Cancer is actually a group of diseases that have one thing in common: groups of cells multiplying out of control.

Normally, about 10 million cells in the body divide every minute under exacting control of the cells' genetic material. This process of cell division is necessary for growth and repair of all body tissues.

But on rare occasions, something goes amiss. A particular control fails, and a cell begins replicating at will, growing, dividing, growing, dividing. The body has mechanisms for spotting and destroying out-of-control cells, but, again on rare occasions, a cluster of such cells escapes detection. Eventually, the cells are growing and dividing so rapidly that they begin causing problems. Depending on where the cells are located, specific symptoms appear.

Doctors diagnose cancer in many ways, but the ultimate diagnosis comes after a sample of the suspect cells is removed from the body and examined under a microscope; cancer cells have a characteristic appearance that distinguishes them from normal cells. Cancers are classified largely according to the site at which they appear—lung cancer, liver cancer, ovarian cancer, and so on.

Some cancers have no connection to diet, or at least none that has been identified as yet. Also, diet is not presumed to be the only factor playing a role in the development of cancer. Nevertheless, as is discussed in the chapters that follow, diet does seem to affect the development of a number of cancers. Those whose development is suspected of being influenced by diet include cancers of the esophagus, stomach, colon and rectum (usually grouped together as colorectal cancer), breast, lung, liver, pancreas, endometrium, ovaries, bladder, and prostate.

Some scientists estimate that 30 to 40 percent of cancers in men and 60 percent of cancers in women are affected by dietary practices. Other researchers have predicted that between 10 and 70 percent of the deaths from cancer are related to diet. This wide range indicates that the scientific evidence is not sufficient to precisely quantify the contribution of diet to the overall risk of cancer. It is also difficult to predict how large the reduction in risk might be if everyone adopted the eating pattern recommended in *Eat for Life*. It is noteworthy, though, that several countries with dietary patterns similar to the pattern recommended in the *Eat for Life* guidelines have about one-half the U.S. mortality rates for cancers associated with diet.

DIABETES

Like cancer, diabetes mellitus—diabetes for short—is a group of diseases with a common biochemical characteristic. In diabetes, the common feature is abnormal metabolism of carbohydrates, particularly glucose. This can lead, over many years, to kidney disease, atherosclerosis, heart attack, stroke, gangrene, and other complications including blindness. In fact, diabetes is the third leading cause of blindness in the United States.

All types of diabetes have something to do with insulin, a hormone produced by special cells in the pancreas, called islets of Langerhans. Insulin is one of several compounds the body uses to control the levels of glucose in the blood. Without insulin, blood sugar levels rise dangerously high. The same thing can happen if the body loses its ability to respond to insulin.

There are two main types of diabetes. The most serious is called insulin-dependent diabetes. In this disorder, the insulin-producing cells of the islets of Langerhans are destroyed, depriving the body of insulin. In most cases, this destruction seems to occur by the body's own hand—cells of the immune system, for some unknown reason, come to see the islets cells as being invaders, and therefore the immune system destroys the cells as it would any foreign object. Diet is not thought to be a cause of this disease.

Insulin-dependent diabetes usually appears well before the age of 40. The only treatment is regular injections of insulin. About 10 percent of all diabetics—about 1.1 million people in the United States—have insulin-dependent diabetes.

The more common form of diabetes is called noninsulin-dependent diabetes. It is closely linked to the resistance to the action of insulin that occurs in obesity. It accounts for about 90 percent of diabetes cases, or nearly 10 million people in the United States. Noninsulin-dependent diabetes usually appears in middle or old age, particularly in people who are overweight. As many as 9 percent of people 65 and older may have this disease. Genetic, environmental, and lifestyle factors can place a person at increased risk for developing noninsulin-dependent diabetes. The most important risk factors are increasing age, family history of diabetes, and obesity—especially fat carried in the abdomen. Researchers have found that fasting blood sugar levels tend to increase as body weight increases, but exactly how these risk factors contribute to the development of noninsulin-dependent diabetes is still the subject of research.

OBESITY

For more than 50 years, life insurance companies have pointed out that greatly increased body weight is associated with an above-average death rate. In the course of investigating why this is so, researchers have developed a number of ways of judging whether people weigh more than they should for optimal health. The two most important factors associated with the risk of developing several chronic diseases are (1) total body fat, most often estimated by the ratio of body weight to height, and (2) distribution of that fat, on the stomach or on the hips and legs.

Two terms are applied to people who weigh more than they should. "Overweight" indicates an excess amount of weight for a given height above some standard. "Obese" indicates an excessively high amount of body fat compared to muscle and bone.

A way of determining whether your weight is appropriate for your height is called the body mass index. Body mass index is calculated as follows: body weight (in kilograms) divided by the square of the height (in meters). It is simple to determine your body mass index by using the nomogram shown in Figure 4.3. The most desirable body mass

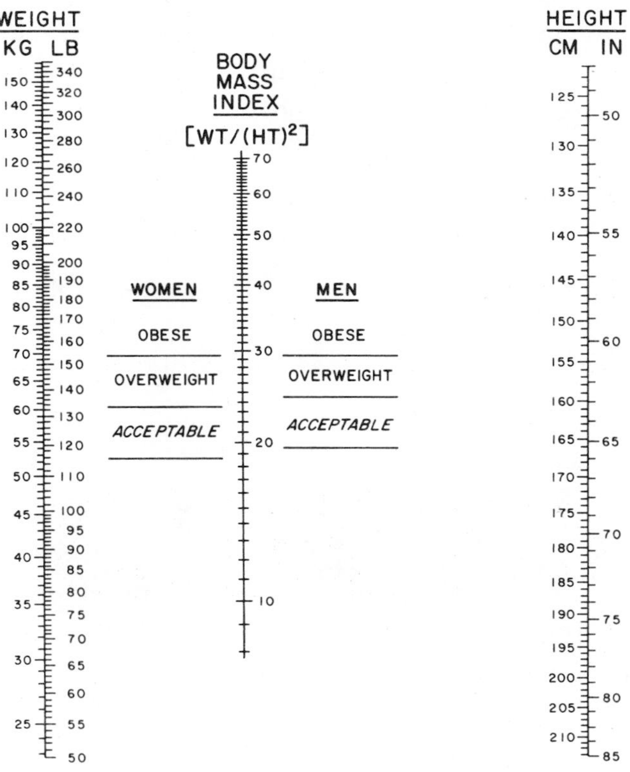

FIGURE 4.3 Nomogram used to determine body mass index. Determine your height without shoes and your weight without clothes. Place a ruler on the nomogram connecting weight on the left with height on the right. The place where it crosses the scale in the center is your body mass index. SOURCE: Copyright 1978, George A. Bray. Used by permission.

index depends on your age, as shown in Table 4.1. A body mass index greater than 30, regardless of age, is considered overweight.

Another way of judging whether you are too fat or too thin is to compare your weight and height to a table based on body mass index and presented in the measurements we are used to using—feet and inches for height and pounds for weight. The weights for heights shown in Table 4.2 are the suggested ranges based on the body mass indexes in Table 4.1. Ranges of weights are given in the table because people of the same height may have equal amounts of body fat but differ in muscle and bone. The higher weights are suggested for people with more muscle and bone. Weights above the range are believed to be unhealthy for most people. Weights slightly below the range may be healthy for some small-boned people but are sometimes linked to health problems, especially if sudden weight loss has occurred.

The distribution of fat on the body is another important variable in the relationship between being overweight and being at risk for chronic diseases. People who deposit fat in the abdominal area are at greater risk of developing strokes,

TABLE 4.1 Desirable Body Mass Indexes by Age Group

Age Group	Body Mass Index
19-24	19-24
25-34	20-25
35-44	21-26
45-54	22-27
55-65	23-28
Over 65	24-29

SOURCE: National Research Council. 1989. *Diet and Health: Implications for Reducing Chronic Disease Risk.* National Academy Press, Washington, D.C.

TABLE 4.2 Suggested Weights for Adults

Height[a]	Weight in Pounds[b,c] 19 to 34 Years	35 Years and Over
5′0"	97-128	108-138
5′1"	101-132	111-143
5′2"	104-137	115-148
5′3"	107-141	119-152
5′4"	111-146	122-157
5′5"	114-150	126-162
5′6"	118-155	130-167
5′7"	121-160	134-172
5′8"	125-164	138-178
5′9"	129-169	142-183
5′10"	132-174	146-188
5′11"	136-179	151-194
6′0"	140-184	155-199
6′1"	144-189	159-205
6′2"	148-195	164-210
6′3"	152-200	168-216
6′4"	156-205	173-222
6′5"	160-211	177-228
6′6"	164-216	182-234

[a]Without shoes.

[b]Without clothes.

[c]The higher weights in the ranges generally apply to men, who tend to have more muscle and bone; the lower weights more often apply to women, who have less muscle and bone.

SOURCE: U.S. Department of Agriculture and U.S. Department of Health and Human Services. 1990. *Dietary Guidelines for Americans*, third edition. U.S. Government Printing Office, Washington, D.C.

coronary heart disease, and diabetes than people who tend to deposit fat in their hips and thighs—called the "femero-gluteal" area. The most common method for determining fat distribution is called the waist-to-hip ratio. You can determine that easily by using the nomogram shown in Figure 4.4.

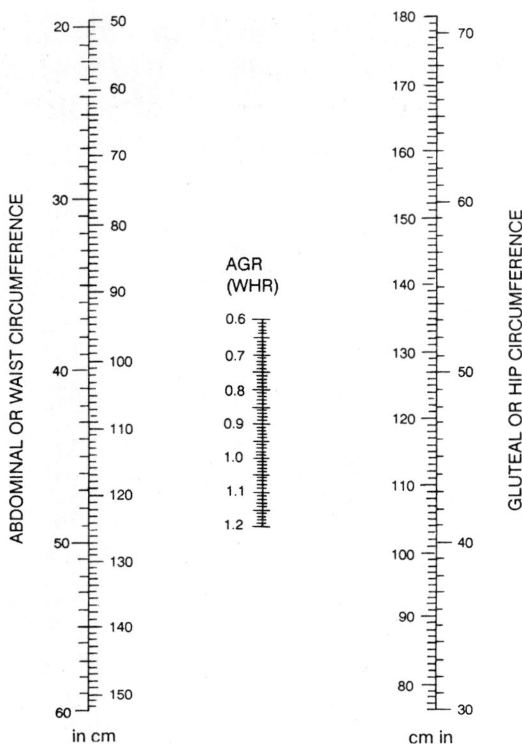

FIGURE 4.4 Nomogram used to determine waist-to-hip ratio. Using a tape measure, measure your waist at the smallest point below your ribs but above your naval. Next, measure your hips at the largest part of your buttocks. Place a ruler on the nomogram connecting size of your waist on the left with size of the hips on the right. Read your abdominal-to-gluteal ratio off the scale in the middle of the nomogram. SOURCE: National Research Council. 1989. *Diet and Health: Implications for Reducing Chronic Disease Risk.* National Academy Press, Washington, D.C.

Waist-to-hip ratios close to or higher than one are linked to a greater risk for several chronic diseases. If your weight for your height is above the suggested range and your waist-to-hip ratio is high, you should consult your doctor to determine a healthy weight for you and set some reasonable weight loss goals.

Approximately 34 million adults in the United States between ages 20 and 74 are overweight, and of these over 12 million are obese. More women are overweight than men, and black people are overweight more often than whites. And, as a whole, the country is gaining weight. With these figures in mind, it should come as no surprise that 27 percent of all men and 46 percent of all women say they are trying to lose weight.

OSTEOPOROSIS

Osteoporosis is a disease in which the bones become fragile. In severe osteoporosis, bone loss can be so bad that bones fracture with very little stress. The most common bones to fracture in osteoporosis are the hip, vertebrae in the spine, forearm, upper arm, pelvis, and ribs.

Bone is composed primarily of calcium, phosphate, and a porous material called collagen. Though bone seems stable, it is constantly being formed and broken down, or reabsorbed. In childhood, adolescence, and young adulthood, more bone is formed than is broken down. In normal adult bones, these two processes are in balance—when one of these activities increases or decreases, so does the other—and the amount of bone remains constant. Then, sometime between ages 35 and 45, bone starts to resorb faster than it forms, so that the amount of bone begins to decrease. In most cases, the difference is very small, less than one-half percent each year.

Women have a special problem, however. For about 8 to 10 years immediately before and after menopause, bone resorbs some 10 times faster than at younger ages. During that period, women can lose between 2 and 5 percent of their bone each year.

About 15 to 20 million people in the United States, the majority of them elderly women, have osteoporosis. People with osteoporosis suffer an estimated 1.3 million bone fractures each year.

GALLSTONES

Gallstones are small, hard pellets that form in the gallbladder. They can block the bile duct, which transports bile from the liver to the small intestine. The major symptom of gallstones is severe pain.

Bile is a mixture of compounds, including cholesterol, that aids digestion by breaking globs of fat in the intestine into tiny droplets, which can then be absorbed into the blood stream. The liver makes bile and stores it in the gallbladder.

There are two major varieties of gallstones: those composed primarily of cholesterol and those made of various pigments derived from hemoglobin, the oxygen-carrying substance of red blood cells. About 80 percent of the gallstones in the United States are the cholesterol variety. They form when bile contains too much cholesterol; the cholesterol then solidifies to form stones.

About 10 percent of all adults in the United States have gallstones. Women are twice as likely as men to develop them. Native Americans are particularly prone to gallstones, with as much as 65 percent of some groups suffering from this disease.

Obesity increases the risk of gallstones by increasing cholesterol secretion into bile. It seems logical that a high cholesterol intake would increase cholesterol secretion into the bile and increase the risk of gallstones, but there is no firm evidence from studies in humans that the concentration of cholesterol in bile is increased by high intakes of cholesterol.

CIRRHOSIS OF THE LIVER

The liver is susceptible to injury from a variety of causes. Cirrhosis of the liver is a chronic disease whose relentless progression destroys normal liver structure and function. Eventually, the liver fails and death results. Cirrhosis may be caused by viral hepatitis, hemachromatosis (a disease in which excess iron accumulates in the liver), obstruction of the biliary system, congestive heart failure, and chronic alcoholism. It is estimated that over half of all deaths from cirrhosis are attributable to alcohol. A good diet, high in carbohydrate and protein, can reduce the impact of the excessive alcohol use that causes cirrhosis.

Deaths from alcohol-induced cirrhosis have declined since 1973, but the disease is still a leading killer. In 1987, cirrhosis killed 26,000 people in the United States, and it was the ninth leading cause of death.

DENTAL CARIES (CAVITIES)

Tooth decay affects more people than any other chronic disease, producing progressive destruction of teeth. Dental caries, more commonly known as cavities, are the end result of tooth decay.

The relationship of diet to dental caries was suspected as early as the fourth century B.C., when Aristotle hypothesized that dental caries were caused by eating sweet figs, which stuck to the teeth. Current evidence indicates that dental caries need two factors to develop—bacteria, particularly *Streptococcus mutans*, and fermentable carbohydrate. The bacteria grow on the surface of the teeth and form plaque, which tends to hold the by-products of the bacterial metabolism close to the tooth surface. The energy source for the oral bacteria is the carbohydrate present in the mouth. As the bacteria process the carbohydrate, they produce acid as a by-product, and that acid corrodes the enamel coating the tooth surface and promotes decay of the underlying tooth.

People in the United States suffer from fewer cavities than at any time in the past, due largely to widespread fluoridation of water supplies and the use of topical fluorides. But tooth decay is still a major problem. The average 18-year-old has had 12 cavities, and the average adult over age 40 has had 29 cavities.

CHAPTER

5

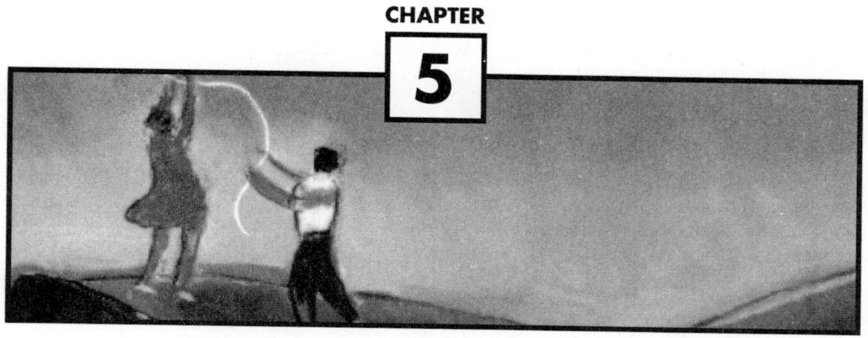

CALORIES, ENERGY BALANCE, AND CHRONIC DISEASES

If you eat too much, or exercise too little, you gain weight. If you gain too much weight, you may put yourself at risk for diabetes or a host of other health problems. Those are warnings doctors have been giving us for a number of years now, and the prescription that usually goes along with that message is to eat less and exercise more. That is sound advice.

But in fact, it has been difficult to pinpoint a connection between the number of calories we consume and the risk we might experience for a particular chronic illness. After all, we do not eat just calories. What we eat are carbohydrates, fats, proteins, and alcohol, and the other nutrients, such as vitamins and minerals, that come along with those calories. Thus two groups of people can eat the same number of calories over many years but have very different diets with a different balance of nutrients.

There is also the matter of energy balance—how does the amount of calories you eat compare with the amount of calories your body uses every day? Again, two groups of people might eat the same number of calories with the same balance of nutrients, but one group leads a very active life, whereas the other has a sedentary lifestyle. Over the years, the more active group will gain less weight than the sedentary group, and this might have an effect on the development of chronic degenerative diseases in the two groups. So it is necessary to look at activity levels, energy balance, changes in body weight, and the composition of the diet, in addition to total calories consumed, when searching for a link between calories and chronic illness.

FUELING UP AND BURNING IT OFF

On average, American men eat about 2360 to 2640 calories a day, and women eat between 1640 and 1800 calories a day. That is about 10 percent less than in 1970.

The number of calories people eat depends on many factors, including their age, activity level, the weather, if they are on a diet, and, for women, if they are pregnant. Take age, for example. Teenage boys eat the greatest number of calories. But as we age, basal metabolism may decline and activity levels may also decrease. The amount we eat drops, so that by the time we reach retirement age we eat a little more than half as much as when we were teens.

There is a fundamental law of nutrition that goes like this: in order to maintain a constant weight, you have to balance the number of calories you eat with the number of calories you burn. To put it simply,

Calories in = Calories out.

If the equation is out of balance, you will either gain or lose weight, depending on which side of the equation is greater. You will not notice any weight change on a day-to-day basis, but you will if the equation remains unbalanced over a period of a week or more. The weight you might gain is stored primarily as fat.

The U.S. population is a good example of what happens when this equation is out of balance. The people in this country may eat 10 percent less than they did in 1970, but, on the whole, the nation has gained weight. The conclusion we can draw from this is that we, as a nation, have become less active over the past two decades. So although we are eating fewer calories than we once were, the rate at which we are burning them has dropped even more. The effect of all this overeating—or underexercising—is that the nation's fat stores have increased.

There are some times when gaining weight and fat is appropriate. Childhood and adolescence are two such times. It is also necessary during pregnancy.

Unless you keep to a regular exercise program as you age, you will find that the amount of fat on your body increases even if your weight does not. If you keep your calorie intake constant, you may have to increase your exercise level as you age to keep a constant weight.

WEIGHT AND CHRONIC ILLNESS

It is not fair to imply that only people who are overweight need to be concerned about their health. In fact, studies of large numbers of people show that it is best—at least from the standpoint of attaining a long life—to be neither too skinny nor too fat. The numbers of deaths and disabilities from heart disease, cancer, diabetes, high blood pressure, gallstones, and osteoporosis all increase in people who are much lighter or heavier than average.

Studying the relationships between body weight and development of chronic diseases is particularly difficult. Some of the relationships are "confounded" by genetic and other factors—for example, thin people may be heavy cigarette smokers, and the smoking may be the true cause of cancer rather than thinness. People's weight may change in the early stages of a disease, prior to its diagnosis, further complicating the study of the relationship of weight to disease.

It has been known for decades that obesity occurs more frequently in some families than in others. Studies of twins suggest that genetics is an important factor in whether people become obese. Because members of a family share meals as well as other habits, identifying the role genetics plays in the development of obesity and the predisposition to chronic diseases is complex. In addition to obesity, there is increasing evidence that patterns of fat distribution are inherited.

Although there is some concern about the effects of being underweight, most research has concentrated on the health effects of being overweight. This is probably because more people in the United States are overweight than underweight. Whatever the reason, the rest of the discussion in this chapter focuses on the problems associated with being overweight or obese. As defined in the previous chapter (page 70), overweight refers to an excess amount of weight for a person of a given height, and obese indicates an excess amount of body fat compared to muscle and bone. Let's look at each disease separately.

Heart Disease

There is little disagreement that the heavier you are, the greater your risk of having a heart attack. People who are 5 to 15 percent overweight have more than twice the number of deaths from heart attacks as people of average weight. For those who are 25 percent or more overweight, the number of fatal heart attacks is 5 times higher than normal.

High Blood Pressure

The evidence is clear: being overweight is associated with having high blood pressure, and losing excess weight usually lowers blood pressure. What is interesting about this, though, is that the effect seems to be related more to body build than to weight itself. People with low waist-to-hip ratios have lower blood pressure than do people with waist-to-hip ratios close to or higher than one.

Diabetes

Excess body fat, which is usually associated with excess body weight, increases the risk of developing noninsulin-dependent diabetes. In fact, the chance of becoming diabetic more than doubles for people who are 20 percent overweight. What is worse, the risk keeps doubling for every additional 20 percent weight gain. For example, if a 5′9" man weighs 190 pounds, instead of the optimal 158 pounds, his risk for developing noninsulin-dependent diabetes doubles. If he gains even more weight, up to 227 pounds, his risk is twice as high again.

As in the case with high blood pressure, noninsulin-dependent diabetes is more common in people who carry their excess weight primarily on the abdomen (those with high waist-to-hip ratios). Being overweight in the hips and thighs (resulting in low waist-to-hip ratio), it seems, does not carry as much of a health penalty as far as diabetes is concerned. This seems particularly true for women.

Losing weight is the most effective therapy for people with noninsulin-dependent diabetes. Study after study has shown that decreasing body weight improves the body's ability to metabolize glucose, the biochemical hallmark of this disease.

Gallstones

The evidence shows clearly that being overweight increases the likelihood of developing gallstones. This is particularly true as a person's age increases. For example, by age 60, nearly one-third of obese women can expect to develop gallbladder disease.

The connection between gallbladder disease and weight stems from the fact that being overweight increases the body's production of cholesterol. With the body making cholesterol, the liver excretes more. This raises the level of cholesterol in bile, which leads to gallstones.

Cancer

The link between cancer and excess weight is not as strong as with the diseases above, but a link does exist. Being overweight increases the risk of endometrial cancer, in particular, although cancers of the gallbladder, bile duct, ovary, breast (in postmenopausal women), cervix, colon, and prostate are also more common in overweight people.

THE DIETING CYCLE

We are a nation that weighs too much, and we seem to know it—a 1985 Gallup poll found that almost 90 percent of U.S. adults believed they weigh too much. As a result, dieting has become a major preoccupation with millions of people in the United States. The same poll found that 31 percent of the women questioned dieted at least once a month, and 16 percent of the women considered themselves perpetual dieters. Other studies have identified even greater numbers of dieters in the U.S. population.

One reason why there are so many people on diets is that most dieters regain the weight they lose. In fact, between 60 and 90 percent of the pounds shed on diets in this country are put back on. To lose these pounds, people go back on diets, and soon a cycle develops—gain, diet, lose, gain, diet, lose, and so on.

The effects of the diet cycle are unclear, but there is some evidence suggesting that it is not a healthy activity. For example, several studies have found that people who gain and lose 10 percent of their weight have a higher risk of developing coronary heart disease than people whose weight remains constant. Repeated cycles of weight gain and weight loss may increase the risk even further. The body may also adjust to the diet cycle by becoming more efficient at using food energy. Thus each attempt to lose weight becomes more difficult. So if you weigh too much now, lose the excess weight by a combination of eating less and exercising much more than you do currently, and if you are not overweight, stay that way.

CHAPTER

6

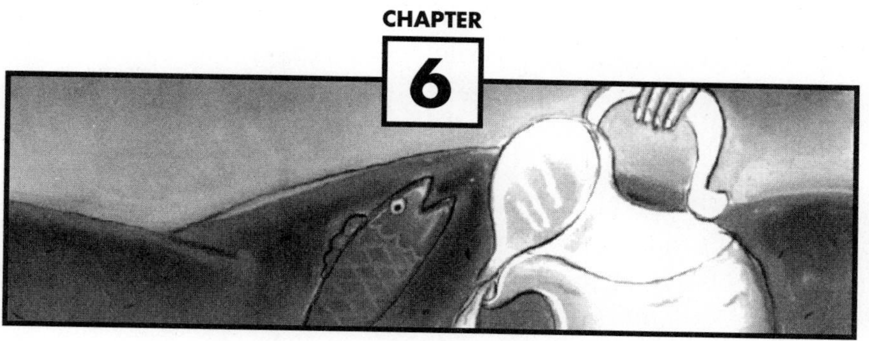

FATS, CHOLESTEROL, AND CHRONIC DISEASES

Without a doubt, fats and cholesterol are the single most important group of nutrients to limit in your diet if you want to help to reduce your risk of chronic disease. Heart disease and cancer, this nation's two leading killers, are linked to diets high in fat, and other chronic health problems may be exacerbated by high-fat diets. And yet our national diet contains as much as one-third more fat than it should.

If your diet is too high in fat—and the chances are good that it is—then read this chapter carefully. It will give you the reasons—and the motivation—to change your diet for the better.

HEART DISEASE

Cornelius de Langen, a Dutch physician working in Java, reported in 1916 that native Indonesians had much less heart disease than did the Dutch colonists living on the island. He associated the natives' healthy hearts with their lower serum cholesterol levels. De Langen also observed that when Indonesians worked as stewards on Dutch passenger ships and ate typical Dutch food, their cholesterol levels soared, and so did their incidence of heart disease.

Although this report lay unnoticed for more than 40 years—it was published in an obscure research journal—it was the first recorded suggestion that diet and serum cholesterol levels in humans were somehow related to heart disease. In the years between then and now, scientists have accumulated an impressive amount of evidence firmly linking the amount and kind of fat and the amount of cholesterol people eat to the risk they stand of having a heart attack. In fact, nowhere is the connection between diet and chronic illness more scientifically firm and convincing than it is with fats and heart disease.

This story of fats and heart disease has three parts. The first reveals the association of high serum cholesterol levels with increased risk of having a heart attack. The second links high saturated fatty acid and cholesterol consumption to high serum cholesterol levels. And the third ties high saturated fatty acid and cholesterol consumption to an increased risk of having a heart attack.

The Case for Lower Serum Cholesterol

Serum cholesterol levels vary widely both among groups of people in various parts of the world and among individuals of those groups. For example, scientists in seven countries worked together to measure serum cholesterol levels in different groups of middle-aged men. The results showed that the average serum cholesterol level of Japanese men was 157 milligrams per deciliter (mg/dl), whereas men living in eastern Finland averaged 262 mg/dl.

There are also large differences among the different peoples of the world in the incidence of heart disease. For example, heart attacks are rare in Mediterranean countries, whereas they are fairly common in Scandinavia.

Because both cholesterol levels and the incidence of heart disease vary greatly among different groups of people, might the two be connected? In other words, do groups of people with high serum cholesterol levels have more heart attacks than populations with low levels? By comparing the rates of heart disease—how many individuals have a heart attack for every 1000 people, for example—with the average serum cholesterol levels among groups of people, scientists have determined that the answer is definitely yes. Populations in which the average serum cholesterol level is less than 180 mg/dl are virtually free of both atherosclerosis and heart disease. In contrast, those groups of people in which the average serum cholesterol level is above 220 mg/dl have high rates of heart attacks.

Further evidence for linking high blood cholesterol levels with the incidence of heart disease comes from many studies of people *within* a particular population group. Since 1948, for example, thousands of volunteers from the city of Framingham, Massachusetts, have been examined every 2 years as part of a comprehensive scientific effort to identify and understand the factors that affect heart health. Results from this study show that, among both men and women, the higher the blood cholesterol level, the greater the risk of developing heart disease. The same relationship was shown in a group of more than 300,000 men across the country aged 35 to 57 years who were medically evaluated as part of a study that came to be known as MR. FIT.

Another way to examine the link between cholesterol level and risk of heart disease is to lower blood cholesterol levels in a large group of volunteers by diet, drugs, or both, and to monitor the number of heart attacks and deaths from heart disease in the group over time. These experiments, known as clinical trials, have enabled scientists to develop the following rule of thumb: each 1 percent reduction in blood cholesterol can be expected to lead to a 2 percent reduction in the risk of heart disease.

As is shown in Chapter 3, not all serum cholesterol is alike. Cholesterol travels through the blood not by itself, but as part of lipoproteins, which are aggregates of lipids and proteins. There are three types of lipoproteins that ferry cholesterol through the blood stream to and from the billions of cells in the body. Low-density lipoproteins (LDLs) carry between 60 and 70 percent of the cholesterol in the blood stream, and high-density lipoproteins (HDLs) carry another 20 to 30 percent. A third lipoprotein, very-low-density lipoproteins (VLDLs), carries the rest, though its main role in the body is to carry triglycerides through the blood stream. In industrial societies, typical LDL-cholesterol values range from 110 to as high as 200 mg/dl or more, and HDL-cholesterol values run from around 30 to near 60 mg/dl.

Once the connection between total serum cholesterol levels and heart disease was firmly established, scientists began wondering if one particular lipoprotein was involved in the relationship. To find the answer, they conducted the same type of studies they did before—they measured lipoprotein levels in different groups of people and determined the rate of heart attacks in those groups.

What these studies showed was that within populations elevated LDL-cholesterol levels were important contributors to high rates of heart disease. Moreover, LDL levels were almost totally responsible for differences among populations in blood cholesterol levels and heart disease risk. What is more, any change in LDL-cholesterol levels was associated with a corresponding change in the incidence of heart attacks. When LDL-cholesterol levels rose, more people had heart attacks.

Another piece of evidence in the case against LDL-cholesterol comes from studies of a disease called familial hypercholesterolemia, FH for short. This is an inherited disease in which there is a defect in the mechanism by which cells take up LDL from the blood stream. Because of that defect, LDL-cholesterol levels are very high in people with FH.

With the less severe (heterozygous) form of FH, in which

the mechanism works at about half its normal rate, LDL-cholesterol levels rise to more than 300 mg/dl. About 1 person in 500 in the United States has heterozygous FH. People affected with heterozygous FH often develop premature heart disease, men in their 40s or earlier, women in their 60s. About 5 percent of men who have heart attacks before they turn 60 have heterozygous FH.

About one in a million people suffer from the very severe (homozygous) form of FH, in which the LDL-removal system is missing entirely. LDL-cholesterol levels soar and can reach 600 to 1000 mg/dl. With very severe FH, heart attacks during the teenage years are common. People with very severe FH rarely survive past age 30.

The story with HDLs is not as clear. Within the United States and most industrialized countries, people with high HDL-cholesterol levels have lower rates of heart disease, and those with low HDL-cholesterol levels are at increased risk of heart disease. Thus, in the popular press and other media, HDL-cholesterol is often referred to as the "good" cholesterol and LDL-cholesterol as the "bad" cholesterol.

The wisdom of lowering total serum cholesterol and LDL-cholesterol levels to prevent heart disease is unquestioned by almost all researchers in cardiovascular diseases. The problem, then, is to determine what, if any, factors in the diet cause total serum cholesterol and LDL-cholesterol to be high in the first place. That brings us to the second part of the story.

The Effects of Fatty Acids (Saturated, Monounsaturated, and Polyunsaturated) and Cholesterol in the Diet

To establish a correlation between diet and serum cholesterol levels, researchers once again studied groups of people. In the early 1950s, scientists examined the eating habits of working-class residents of Naples, in southern Italy. The great bulk of these people's diets consisted of bread and pasta, with only 20 percent of their calories coming from fat. They ate cheese and meat in small amounts, used olive oil sparingly, and ate no butter at all. Their serum cholesterol levels averaged a healthy 172 mg/dl.

At about the same time, other investigators examined a group of apparently healthy male factory workers who had lived their adult lives in the United States but whose parents had been born near Naples. These men got about 43 percent of their calories from fat—most of it from animal fats—and their average serum cholesterol level was 239 mg/dl.

Similar studies have shown consistently the same results: People who get a big share of their calories from fats, particularly animal fats with a high proportion of saturated fatty acids, have higher total cholesterol and LDL-cholesterol levels than people who eat diets that are relatively low in fat, particularly saturated fatty acids.

The story is a little more complicated than this, however, for not all saturated fatty acids have the same cholesterol-raising effect. In experiments that began in the late 1950s, scientists fed volunteers foods that were rich in saturated fatty acids. All the foods but one—cocoa butter—had the predicted effect of raising serum cholesterol levels. The major saturated fatty acid in cocoa butter is stearic acid, which contains 18 carbon atoms.

Other studies confirmed this observation and, in addition, showed that saturated fatty acids with 10 or fewer carbon atoms have no effect on serum cholesterol levels either. These studies have shown that palmitic acid (16 carbon atoms) and myristic acid (14 carbon atoms) are the major cholesterol-raising saturated fatty acids. Lauric acid (12 carbon atoms) probably also raises serum cholesterol levels.

Scientists suspect that these saturated fatty acids interfere somehow with the LDL-removal system of the body's cells. As a result, LDL-cholesterol accumulates in the blood stream and eventually deposits its cholesterol onto atherosclerotic plaques in arteries. In a way, these saturated fatty acids mimic the effects of FH, the inherited disorder that causes LDL-cholesterol to rise.

Now what about cholesterol itself: Does eating a lot of cholesterol raise the levels of LDL-cholesterol? The answer is yes, although the LDL-raising effect of dietary cholesterol is not as large as that of the cholesterol-raising saturated fatty acids. On average, eating 200 mg of cholesterol per 2000 calories raises LDL-cholesterol levels by about 8 to 10 mg/dl above what they would be without eating any cholesterol; eating larger amounts of cholesterol produces a further rise. So if you now eat 750 mg of cholesterol a day, you should be able to cut your LDL-cholesterol levels simply by lowering the amount of cholesterol you eat to 250 mg a day. As a result, you might also reduce significantly your risk of having a heart attack.

The foregoing discussion is based on how groups of people respond to different levels of dietary cholesterol. Within the group, however, individuals vary in how responsive they are. Some people are resistant to the LDL-raising effect of dietary cholesterol, whereas others—at least one-third of the U.S. population—are quite sensitive. Unfortunately, it is not feasible on a national scale to find out who is sensitive to dietary cholesterol and who is not; testing cholesterol responsiveness involves eating a controlled diet for weeks and analyzing several blood samples. So until the day comes that we can take a cholesterol response test as easily as we can a serum cholesterol test, we should all try to reduce our cholesterol levels by not eating a large amount of foods that are high in cholesterol.

Whereas cholesterol and saturated fatty acids in the diet have been shown to have detrimental effects, monounsaturated and polyunsaturated fatty acids in the diet are a different story.

In the 1950s, researchers observed that diets containing various vegetable oils reduced serum cholesterol levels when compared with animal fats, regardless of dietary cholesterol intake. These findings have been widely confirmed. It has also been shown that replacing saturated fatty acids with monounsaturated or polyunsaturated fatty acids causes LDL-cholesterol levels to drop substantially. With monounsaturated fatty acids, there is no effect on HDL-cholesterol levels, whereas with polyunsaturated fatty acids there is a tendency for HDL-cholesterol levels to fall as well.

These findings have important practical implications. You do not need to lower your fat intake drastically to reduce your serum cholesterol and LDL-cholesterol levels. Rather, reduce your intake of saturated fatty acids by replacing them in part with carbohydrates and in part with vegetable oils rich in monounsaturated fatty acids (such as olive and canola oil). These measures will help to keep your diet palatable and interesting.

Studies in animals and the study in two groups of veterans mentioned in the next section suggest that diets high in polyunsaturated fatty acids may be linked to other chronic diseases. Because there are no human diets that are naturally high in polyunsaturated fatty acids and because information is lacking about the long-term health consequences of such a diet, you should not increase your intake of polyunsaturated fatty acids over what is now in the U.S. diet (an average of 7 percent of daily calories).

Saturated Fatty Acids and Heart Disease

There is a famous truth in mathematics that states: If A equals B, and B equals C, then A must equal C.

Applying the same logic to nutrition, we would arrive at the conclusion that eating a lot of saturated fatty acids raises the risk of developing heart disease. For if diets high in saturated fatty acids "equal" high total serum cholesterol and high LDL-cholesterol, and if high serum and LDL-cholesterol "equal" high incidence of heart disease, then it must be true that diets high in saturated fatty acids "equal" high incidence of heart disease.

Scientists, however, are rarely content to prove such important connections using mathematical logic, and so they turned once again to examining the rates of heart disease in various populations around the world. They found that there is indeed a strong association between diets high in saturated fatty acids and a high incidence of heart attacks.

These studies also showed clearly that saturated fatty acids could explain the association. On the island of Crete, for example, many of the residents consumed a diet that contained as much as 40 percent of their daily calories as fat, and yet they suffered very little from heart disease. The investigators concluded that the relationship was probably due to the low level of saturated fatty acids, which accounted for only 8 percent of the daily calories in Crete, while monounsaturated fatty acids made up 29 percent of the calories.

In another study, designed as a controlled dietary trial, researchers compared the incidence of heart attacks in two groups of veterans who were randomly assigned to two diets. The men in both groups ate diets in which fat provided 40 percent of the calories. But while one group ate a typical U.S. diet high in saturated fatty acids, the other group ate a diet in which monounsaturated fatty acids and polyunsaturated fatty acids each accounted for about 15 percent of the total calories and saturated fatty acids were reduced to approximately 10 percent of total calories. Almost immediately, the serum cholesterol levels in the group with the diet low in saturated fatty acids dropped nearly 13 percent. The number of deaths from heart disease in this group fell 31 percent.

HIGH BLOOD PRESSURE

People who follow a strict vegetarian diet—no meat, poultry, fish, eggs, or dairy products—tend to have lower blood pressure than those who eat a typical U.S. diet. Since strict vegetarians eat more monounsaturated fatty acids and polyunsaturated fatty acids, and less total fat, saturated fatty acids, and cholesterol, it is reasonable to suspect that dietary fat may have something to do with developing hypertension. Other factors that help keep the blood pressures of strict vegetarians low are their tendencies to refrain from smoking, to be within their ideal weights, and to get regular exercise.

What a number of studies show is that the total amount of fat in the diet does not seem to affect blood pressure. In some studies, however, the levels of saturated fatty acids and of linoleic acid seem to have a modest effect. People living in rural Finland, for example, eat more saturated fatty acids and on average have higher blood pressures than rural residents of the United States and Italy. When volunteers eat special diets containing various amounts of saturated fatty acids and polyunsaturated fatty acids, those people eating a diet in which the amounts of saturated fatty acids and polyunsaturated fatty acids were equal have lower blood pressures, on average, than those eating food high in saturated fatty acids and low in polyunsaturated fatty acids.

Again, these results do not mean you should eat more polyunsaturated fatty acids and less saturated fatty acids to lower your blood pressure. Rather, you should eat less saturated fatty acids while keeping the amount of polyunsaturated fatty acids in your diet about constant at about 7 percent of your daily calories. Polyunsaturated fatty acid intake should not exceed 10 percent of caloric intake.

CANCER

Eating a diet high in fat can increase the risk of developing cancer, particularly cancers of the colon and breast. Studies of cancer rates and eating habits among the different people of the world show a consistent relationship between high-fat diets and high overall cancer rates. None of these studies, though, are as conclusive as those linking high-fat diets to heart disease.

Studies of the relationship of dietary fat to the development of cancer are confounded by several factors. High-fat diets tend to be low in complex carbohydrates, fiber, and fruits and vegetables—all thought to help prevent cancer. High-fat diets are also associated with higher caloric intakes and obesity, factors that are suspected to encourage the development of some cancers.

It has been difficult, too, to pinpoint any connections between dietary fat and specific cancers, or between specific types of fat and cancer. Studies of breast cancer, for example, tend to support a weak link between dietary fat and the risk of developing breast cancer. Some of these studies also single out saturated fatty acids, while others do not.

Why the inconsistencies? One reason might be that the amount of fat eaten early in life may have a greater influence on breast cancer risk than fat eaten as adults. Therefore, when adults lower their fat intake, it might take years to show a beneficial effect on cancer rates.

Another plausible explanation for the less-than-conclusive results of population studies is that it is difficult to reconstruct a person's diet over the many years before cancer develops. In addition, population studies are often not sensitive enough to detect links between diet and disease. Such confusion would help to obscure any diet-cancer link. These last two problems are not specific to studies of breast cancer.

Diets high in fat, particularly saturated fatty acids, appear to increase the risk of developing colon and rectal cancers. There is also evidence of a link between diets high in animal fat and prostate cancer. One study has shown that endometrial cancer occurs more often in parts of the world where the residents eat a high-fat diet, but other studies have been inconclusive. Overall, the evidence is strong enough to support a recommendation to eat less fat in order to reduce the risk of cancer.

OTHER CHRONIC DEGENERATIVE DISEASES

There is little conclusive evidence that dietary fat plays a role in causing any chronic diseases other than heart disease and cancer. Some studies suggest that lowering fat intake, as well as reducing alcohol intake, may allow obese and overweight people to lose weight, but this may be mainly an effect of lowering the total number of calories in the diet.

Gallstones are more common in people who eat diets high in fat and who are overweight or obese, but weight seems to be the major contributing factor. Thus if a low-fat diet can enable overweight and obese people to lose weight, such a diet will indirectly reduce the risk for gallbladder disease.

CHILDREN: A SPECIAL CASE?

The evidence is clear that U.S. adults need to reduce the amount of fat, particularly saturated fatty acids, that they eat. It appears that children eat too much fat as well. Because diet and exercise patterns are established in youth, it is particularly important for parents to move their children away from a high-fat diet and sedentary life and into a low-fat diet and an active life.

Infants and toddlers, that is, children who are less than two years old, are a special case, however. An infant's diet is high in cholesterol and fat—about half the calories in mother's milk come from fat, and saturated fatty acids make up almost half of those calories. Cow's milk and infant formula are also high in fat, but they contain a different mix of fatty acids than mother's milk. Cow's milk, for example, has more saturated fatty acids, less monounsaturated fatty acids, and much less polyunsaturated fatty acids. In contrast, infant formulas are higher in polyunsaturated fatty acids, but contain virtually no cholesterol.

Infants respond to high-fat, high-cholesterol milk in the same way that adults would—their serum cholesterol levels are raised. But most health experts believe this should be no cause for concern. For one thing, children breastfeed or take formula for only a short period of time, so the high cholesterol level probably has no lasting effects. Perhaps even more important, however, breast milk, in particular, meets other nutritional needs of infants. Thus, parents should not try to reduce the amount of fat their infants and toddlers eat.

But that is not the case with children once they start eating the same foods as adults. Several studies of children's eating habits show that U.S. school-age children's diets contain an average of 38 percent fat—much of it saturated fatty acids—and 300 mg of cholesterol. As a result, children in the United States have relatively high serum cholesterol levels.

The consequences of having high serum cholesterol as a child are not yet clear, but two pieces of evidence suggest that the outcome may not be good. For one thing, children with high cholesterol levels tend to become teenagers and young adults with high cholesterol. In addition, doctors have found that significant numbers of young adults already have detectable atherosclerosis. Therefore it seems that children have as much to gain from reducing their fat intake as do adults.

Some people have questioned the safety of tampering with our children's diets. After all, our children are far healthier today than they were at the beginning of this century, thanks in part to improved nutrition. But many studies show that a low-fat diet is safe for children. These studies show, too, that there is no need for anyone over the age of two to get more than 30 percent of their calories from fat.

CHAPTER

7

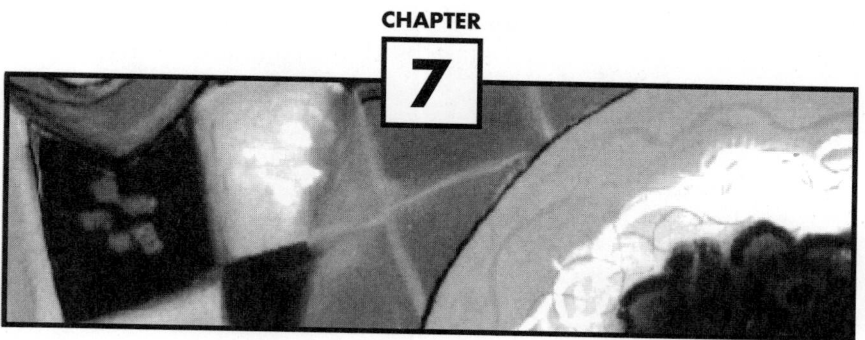

PROTEIN, CARBOHYDRATES, AND CHRONIC DISEASES

As nutrients, protein is overemphasized and carbohydrates are underrated in terms of their importance in our diets. Most people in the United States now eat more protein than their bodies need, and, somehow, carbohydrate-rich foods such as potatoes and bread have gotten a bad name for being fattening. Yet protein from animal sources often comes in foods that contain significant amounts of saturated fatty acids. And the only carbohydrate-rich foods that are truly fattening are those laden with fats and added sugar, such as pastries, cookies, and baked potatoes heaped with sour cream.

In fact, there is some evidence that diets high in carbohydrates may help reduce the risk of heart disease. Thus the *Eat for Life* guidelines suggest not to eat any more protein than you already do and to increase the amount of carbohydrates you eat to compensate for the lower amount of fat that your diet will contain.

This chapter presents the evidence that increasing the proportion of carbohydrates in the usual American eating pattern at the expense of fat will tend to lower chronic disease risk. It also discusses some of the health claims made for dietary fiber, a group of substances that are made up mostly of complex carbohydrates.

PROTEIN

Heart Disease

Health experts have suspected that protein from animal sources contributes to an increased risk of heart disease, since people who eat diets high in animal protein usually suffer more heart attacks than people who get their protein mainly from plant sources. But it may be that animal protein is not to blame at all. Any association of protein intake with high cholesterol levels and high cardiovascular disease risk in populations is largely explained by the levels of saturated fatty acids in the protein-containing food. Many foods of animal origin, such as meats and dairy products, contain saturated fatty acids. So in all likelihood it is the fat content of diets high in animal protein that causes an increase in heart attacks, not the protein.

There is evidence, though, that vegetable protein may exert some beneficial effects that animal protein does not. In one experiment, for example, volunteers with high serum cholesterol levels ate diets in which all their protein came from soybeans. Both serum cholesterol and LDL-cholesterol levels dropped substantially in this group.

Cancer

As with heart disease, diets that are high in animal products appear to increase the risk for cancer. But, also as with heart disease, this seems to be more a factor of the animal fat associated with animal protein than the protein itself.

Osteoporosis

There seems to be little increased risk of osteoporosis from eating a high-protein diet. Consumption of large amounts of purified animal protein is associated with calcium loss in the urine. But few of us increase the amount of protein we eat by adding purified animal protein to our diets. Instead, we eat protein-containing foods like meat, which contains significant amounts of phosphorus, and phosphorus seems to minimize any effect protein has on calcium excretion. Therefore you do not need to worry that eating meat increases your chances of developing osteoporosis.

CARBOHYDRATES

Dental Caries

There is little doubt that simple carbohydrates, otherwise known as sugars, are involved in causing dental caries. This is particularly true when sugar is eaten between meals and as part of sticky foods. It also appears, though, that most carbohydrates, as least to some extent, can cause cavities.

Carbohydrates play a role in tooth decay by acting as an energy source for the bacteria that live in the mouth. These bacteria break down sugar and produce acids that can remove minerals from teeth. The body has mechanisms for putting those minerals back into teeth, but once the bacteria get a good hold on a particular tooth, the microbe can break down a tooth's surface faster than the body can rebuild it. Eventually, if nothing is done to disturb acid production by the bacteria, a cavity develops.

Not all carbohydrates are as effective in feeding this process. Sucrose—common table sugar—appears to be the worst offender. Fructose, a sugar in honey and fruit, is not as bad, but it, too, serves as a good energy source for mouth bacteria. Foods rich in complex carbohydrates and fiber may actually help protect against cavities. Chewing them stimulates the flow of saliva and neutralizes the acids produced by the bacteria.

Developing tooth decay is not simply a matter of how much sugar you might eat, but when and with what foods. For example, eating cheese right after eating sugar seems to neutralize the acid that mouth bacteria produce.

Experiments show, too, that it is not the amount of sugar you consume, but how you eat it—sucking on hard candy all day would promote tooth decay more than eating one large piece of rock candy in 15 minutes. Soft drinks are less apt to promote cavities than hard candies—sugar in solid foods promotes cavities more than does sugar in liquid foods.

Noninsulin-Dependent Diabetes

Contrary to popular belief, diets high in carbohydrates are not associated with an increased risk of developing noninsulin-dependent diabetes. In fact, the opposite seems to be true: The risk of developing noninsulin-dependent diabetes decreases as the amount of calories from carbohydrates increases.

Compared to low-carbohydrate diets, diets high in carbohydrates improve the body's sensitivity to insulin. Therefore, many physicians recommend that their patients with noninsulin-dependent diabetes switch to a high-carbohydrate, low-fat diet. Such a switch seems to reduce the number of symptoms these people experience, although the best course of action for this disease is to lose weight. Another reason why a high-carbohydrate, low-fat diet may also benefit people with noninsulin-dependent diabetes is because it reduces their risk of developing heart disease, a major cause of death among people with diabetes.

FIBER

The word "fiber" actually describes many different mixtures of carbohydrates and other large molecules present in almost all plant foods. An eating pattern that is high in fiber is high in vegetables, whole-grain products, fruits, and legumes (beans and peas) and low in animal products. A high-fiber eating pattern is high in complex carbohydrates and relatively low in fat.

Because the mix called "fiber" may be made up of many different substances, depending on the source, it has been difficult to clarify the role of fiber in health and disease. What evidence we have appears to be positive.

There are two kinds of fiber: insoluble fiber, which exerts its effects primarily in the digestive system, and soluble fiber, which has effects on substances in the blood stream. Diets high in both kinds of fiber tend to be bulky, and since fiber itself does not contribute calories, foods high in fiber tend to contain fewer calories in the same volume of food. These characteristics of high-fiber diets may help assuage hunger and thus contribute to weight loss.

Fiber also stimulates the liver to produce more bile, thus aiding digestion. Insoluble fiber also causes digested food to pass through the intestines more quickly, thus contributing to "regularity" and reducing the length of time the gut lining is in contact with any potentially harmful substances contained in the digested food.

Heart Disease

People who eat diets that are high in fiber have significantly lower serum cholesterol and higher HDL-cholesterol levels than people who eat low-fiber diets. Comparisons of cholesterol levels among populations eating different levels of fiber—complete vegetarians, lacto-ovovegetarians, and nonvegetarians—showed that the high-fiber-consuming vegetarians had the lowest serum cholesterols, followed by the lacto-ovovegetarians, and finally the lowest-fiber-consuming nonvegetarians.

Studies show that it is soluble fibers (like those in fresh fruits, vegetables, and beans) rather than insoluble fibers (like those in the bran of wheat) that appear to have an effect on serum cholesterol. Indeed, studies have shown that guar gum, pectin, and oat bran—all soluble fibers—seem to lower LDL-cholesterol. The connection between high-fiber diets and fewer heart attacks is less clear. Some studies suggest that it is the low fat content of high-fiber diets that reduces the risk of heart disease. Other studies, however, show that eating a diet high in fiber, regardless of its fat content, reduces the risk of developing heart disease. For now, the question of whether or not a high-fiber diet will protect you against heart disease remains unanswered. What is clear, though, is that a high-fiber eating pattern will help to lower your serum cholesterol and also help to lower your risk of heart disease.

Cancer

Cancer of the large intestine is rare in Africa, where people eat diets high in fiber, which suggests that fiber may protect against colon cancer. But studies of groups of people who differ in the amount of fiber they eat have not proven this idea true. The conflicting results—some studies showed a protective effect and others showed no effect—may stem from the problems of comparing fibers from different sources.

Other Chronic Diseases

Fiber, according to what you might read in magazines and newspapers, seems to be the one dietary component that affords some protection against nearly every chronic disease known. While that may, indeed, prove to be true, the scientific evidence so far is sketchy. Various studies have shown, for instance, that diets high in fiber may benefit people with noninsulin-dependent diabetes and may even help prevent this disease. Other studies have suggested that high-fiber diets can lower high blood pressure and reduce the chances of developing gallstones. But all of these studies focus on fiber-rich diets, not fiber itself. It may be that other components of these diets are at work, perhaps in combination with fiber, in lowering the risk for these chronic diseases.

Can Too Much Fiber Be Bad?

Some health experts have raised the concern that high-fiber diets may make it difficult for the body to absorb important minerals from the digestive system. This does not appear to happen, however. For example, vegetarians eating high-fiber diets have normal levels of iron, zinc, copper, and selenium in their bodies. Similarly, the levels of iron, calcium, and magnesium are the same in people with diabetes who eat a high-fiber diet and in those who eat the average U.S. diet. The conclusion seems to be that there is little evidence that high-fiber diets alone will produce a mineral deficiency in people who otherwise consume a balanced diet.

You should be aware, however, that switching abruptly from a low-fiber diet to one high in fiber may make you feel bloated and nauseous and may cause flatulence. This is particularly true if the increased fiber comes from wheat bran and guar gum. These effects are temporary, though, and diminish after a few weeks. On the plus side, a high-fiber diet reduces constipation and contributes to more regular bowel movements. You are likely to be more comfortable if you gradually increase your intake of fiber-rich foods.

One final word on fiber—do not start taking fiber supplements based on what you have read here. There is an impressive amount of evidence showing the beneficial effects of eating a diet containing a large amount of fruits and vegetables (i.e., fiber-containing foods), and relatively low levels of meat and fatty products. We do not know, yet, whether the benefits of such a diet are the result of the large amounts of fiber and carbohydrates, low amounts of fat, other protective factors in plants, a combination of the three, or some other dietary factor. Therefore, although it is desirable to eat a diet containing fiber-rich foods, it is not necessary to take fiber supplements unless specifically advised to do so by your doctor.

CHAPTER

8

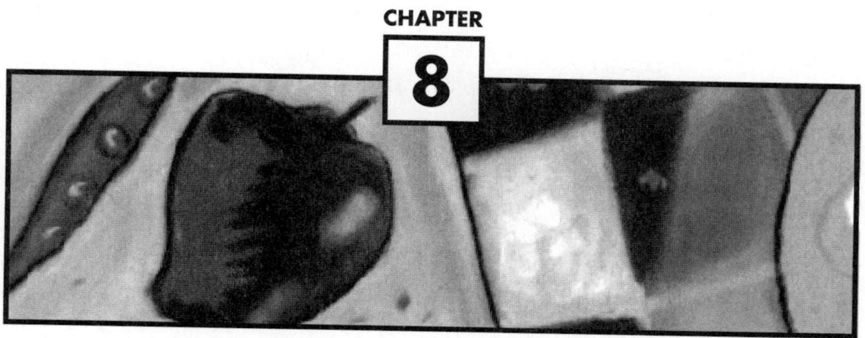

VITAMINS, MINERALS, AND CHRONIC DISEASES

Vitamins and minerals are a diverse group of substances that play an enormous number of roles in the body. Compared to proteins, carbohydrates, and fats, the body needs very small amounts of these nutrients to remain in good working order, and yet eating too little or too much of them can be physically devastating.

Today, it is rare for people in the United States to suffer from severe vitamin or mineral deficiencies; those disorders, such as rickets and pellagra, are not the subject of this chapter. Instead, we are more likely to consume too much of some minerals and not quite enough of other minerals and vitamins. One of the goals of the *Eat for Life* guidelines, in fact, is to ensure that you get adequate amounts of these nutrients as part of your usual eating pattern. Therefore by simply following the *Eat for Life* guidelines, you will be eating foods that provide you with sufficient vitamins and minerals. This chapter reviews the evidence linking slight deficiencies or excesses of vitamins and minerals to a number of chronic diseases.

VITAMINS

In this section only those vitamins thought to have some connection with chronic disease are discussed.

Vitamin A

The body gets vitamin A from two different sets of chemicals—retinoids and carotenoids. Vitamin A itself is the compound retinol. It and the similar compounds belonging to the retinoid family occur only in foods of animal origin, such as liver, butter, milk, and egg yolks.

The body can also make vitamin A from select members of the carotenoid family of compounds, which are present in dark-green, leafy vegetables and in yellow and orange vegetables and fruits. The most common carotenoid is beta-carotene. Enzymes in the small intestine split beta-carotene (and certain closely related carotenoids) to produce vitamin A.

Food labels and nutritional tables state the "vitamin A activity" in a particular product or food. This value, stated in international units (I.U.), reflects how much vitamin A in total—vitamin A, other retinoids, and carotenoids that yield the vitamin—the body gets from that product. Another unit for measuring vitamin A activity is the retinol equivalent (RE). The relationship between REs and I.U.s of vitamin A depends on the form of the vitamin. For example, 1 RE equals 3.33 I.U. of retinol or 10 I.U. of beta-carotene.

Early epidemiologic studies of diet and cancer focused on foods with vitamin A activity but did not distinguish between the retinoids and the carotenoids. For example, studies found that cigarette smokers who eat a large amount of foods containing vitamin A activity were less likely to develop lung cancer than people who did not eat such foods. Later, researchers showed that it was the carotenoids, and not vitamin A or other retinoids, that exerted the protective effect. Because of the results, doctors are now trying to determine the effect of dietary beta-carotene supplements on lung cancer. The results of these experiments will be some time in coming.

Similar tests are under way in which scientists want to determine if beta-carotene can prevent other cancers from developing. These experiments were prompted by studies showing that people who ate foods rich in beta-carotene had lower rates of a variety of cancers, including those of the stomach, cervix, bladder, mouth, larynx, and esophagus. None of these studies were particularly convincing, however, and so we must await the results of further research before we proclaim beta-carotene an all-around cancer preventative.

Retinol and other retinoids have been shown to be protective against experimentally induced cancers in several animal species. The role of retinoids in the prevention or treatment of human cancer is being tested in studies being conducted in a number of different locations.

Vitamin C

Vitamin C (also known as ascorbic acid), perhaps more than any other vitamin, has long been a favorite of those claiming that certain nutrients can prevent cancer and other chronic diseases. The problem with most studies of vitamin C as a cancer preventative is that foods rich in vitamin C also contain other nutrients—fiber, vitamin A, and vitamin E, for example—that may have a protective effect as well.

What researchers have found so far is that vitamin-C-containing foods, and possibly vitamin C itself, may protect against some cancers. The strongest evidence for such a protective effect is with stomach cancer; the evidence for cancer of the esophagus is not as convincing.

Vitamin C may also play a role in preventing atherosclerosis, although, again, the studies conducted so far have not been particularly convincing. One study found that people with atherosclerosis had low levels of vitamin C in their blood stream, implying that these people were not getting enough of the vitamin in their diets. In another study, volunteers under age 25 who took 1-gram (g) supplements of vitamin C [well above the recommended levels] each day experienced a drop in their serum cholesterol levels. Older volunteers did not show a consistent change in cholesterol level when they took the vitamin C supplement.

On the whole, the evidence presented above does not warrant taking large doses of vitamin C as a supplement. Nevertheless, it is a good idea to include plenty of food rich in vitamin C in your diet.

Vitamin D

Vitamin D's main purpose is to increase the amount of calcium in the body and thus increase the amount of calcium that goes into bones. The vitamin does this in several ways. First, it boosts the intestine's ability to absorb calcium from digested food. In addition, vitamin D improves the kidneys' capacity to recycle calcium that might otherwise pass from the blood stream into the urine.

Thus it is not surprising that scientists have been looking for a connection between inadequate consumption of vitamin D and two bone diseases, osteoporosis and osteomalacia. Osteoporosis is a disease in which the bones lose mass (both minerals and bone matrix), eventually leading to fractures in older people. Osteomalacia is a disorder of adults in which bones become soft because the ratio of mineral to the protein component of bone decreases. This disease is known as rickets when it occurs in children.

In countries with limited sunlight, or where the people dress in a fashion that reduces exposure to sunlight, there is a higher incidence of osteomalacia and rickets than in places where the inhabitants get plenty of sunshine (or vitamin D from food). Northern China, Great Britain, Scandinavia, countries in the Middle East, and other Muslim countries are among those in which osteomalacia is relatively common.

With osteoporosis the situation is more complicated. It is true that women with osteoporosis have lower levels of vitamin D in their blood than women who do not have the disease. However, efforts to treat osteoporosis with the active form of vitamin D have had mixed results. On the one hand, people who receive the treatment show higher levels of calcium in their blood stream, suggesting that their intestines are more efficient at absorbing calcium from food sources. But despite the higher calcium levels in their blood, the treated group's bones do not contain any more calcium than the bones of people with osteoporosis who are not treated with the vitamin.

Vitamin E

Countless newspaper and magazine stories have touted vitamin E supplements as an effective cancer preventive. However, study after study has failed to find any connection between the amount of vitamin E people eat and their risk for cancer. A few studies have found, however, that if selenium consumption is low, then an inadequate amount of vitamin E can increase the risk of breast and lung cancer.

Riboflavin

For over 30 years, scientists have suspected that low levels of riboflavin may increase the risk of developing cancer of the esophagus. Although no definite connection has ever been made, a number of studies suggest that low levels of riboflavin may allow alcohol or substances in chewing tobacco to promote cancer of the esophagus. So, if you drink alcoholic beverages or chew tobacco, make sure your diet contains some riboflavin-rich foods.

Vitamins and Alcoholism

One of the most consistent findings in research on vitamins is that alcoholics are often deficient in many of these nutrients, including vitamins B_6 and B_{12}, thiamin, riboflavin, niacin, and folacin. In fact, alcoholism is probably the number one cause of most cases of multivitamin deficiency in the United States.

In many instances, vitamin deficiencies are tied to the liver damage that develops after years of heavy drinking. In other cases, alcohol damages the intestines' ability to absorb vitamins from the digested food. And then there is the problem of alcoholic malnutrition: alcoholics tend to get a large share of their calories from alcohol, and they do not eat enough of other foods. As a result, their consumption of many vitamins is very inadequate.

MINERALS

Food contains dozens of minerals in varying amounts. Some of these are known to be essential nutrients. Others are toxic, although in amounts that greatly exceed the amount consumed in a normal U.S. diet. And then there are those that just happen to be present in the foods we eat, serving no apparent purpose but doing no apparent harm. Every once in a while, new research shows that some mineral in this latter group is, in fact, essential in very small amounts, or perhaps toxic in amounts larger than we consume ordinarily.

The discussion in this section skips those minerals in which there is no strong connection between consumption and disease as well as those minerals, such as lead and cadmium, that are toxic in large amounts but are not related to chronic diseases at the levels found in food.

Calcium

For many people in the United States, getting enough calcium is a constant challenge. In general, dairy products are very good sources of calcium. In fact, it is difficult to get adequate levels of this mineral without eating these foods.

Low calcium intake is almost certainly connected to osteoporosis. Human bones reach their maximum mass at about age 25 to 30, so it is imperative that children, teenagers, and young adults eat calcium-rich foods. To achieve peak bone mass, the Committee on Diet and Health recommended that adolescents and young adults 11 to 25 years of age consume about 1200 mg of calcium per day. Once bones reach their maximum mass, they stabilize for the next 10 to 20 years, and the need for this mineral drops to 800 mg/day. Then, between ages 35 and 45, bones start losing their calcium (even if the diet is high in calcium), a process that accelerates in women immediately before and after menopause.

If calcium intake is low during childhood and adolescence, bones will not develop to the fullest extent possible, which later in life could translate into weaker bones and eventually osteoporosis. In a survey of women in 12 countries, researchers found a direct relationship between high calcium consumption and low risk for osteoporosis. Women in Finland consumed the largest amount of calcium—about 1300 mg/day—and had the lowest number of fractures. In contrast, among Japanese women, who ate the lowest amount of calcium—a mere 400 mg/day—fractures were the most common.

One way of countering bone loss as we age might be to take calcium supplements. However, tests conducted to date have been disappointing. In fact, the most effective way for women at risk for developing osteoporosis to avoid this disorder is to receive estrogen treatment after menopause, which virtually stops bone loss completely. For women who cannot or will not take estrogen therapy, calcium plus vitamin D supplementation may slow bone loss to a degree.

Fluoride

In the late 1930s, scientists began studies that would lead to one of the most significant advances in public health. These researchers were investigating whether there was a relationship between the fluoride content of water and the prevalence of tooth decay. There was, and since 1949 communities across the country have added fluoride to drinking water, helping to produce a dramatic reduction in the number of cavities we now develop.

How good is fluoride at preventing cavities? Children who live for a few years in a community with optimal fluoride levels in drinking water have up to 60 percent fewer cavities. Despite the unparalleled success of fluoridation, more than 45 percent of the U.S. population still drinks water with less than optimal levels of fluoride. To address this need, the American Dental Association, the American Academy of Pediatrics, and the American Academy of Pediatric Dentistry have issued guidelines, shown in Figure 8.1, for giving children fluoride supplements.

If you think you or your children do not receive an adequate amount of fluoride in your drinking water, see your physician. It is important not to take too much fluoride because this can actually damage teeth.

Iron

Iron is an essential element, present in all body cells. It is part of the hemoglobin found in red blood cells, where its main function is to carry oxygen in the blood stream. It is also an important component of certain enzymes. Good food sources of iron include red meats, poultry, fish, whole and enriched grain products, and dark-green leafy vegetables.

Iron-deficiency anemia is the most obvious disorder re-

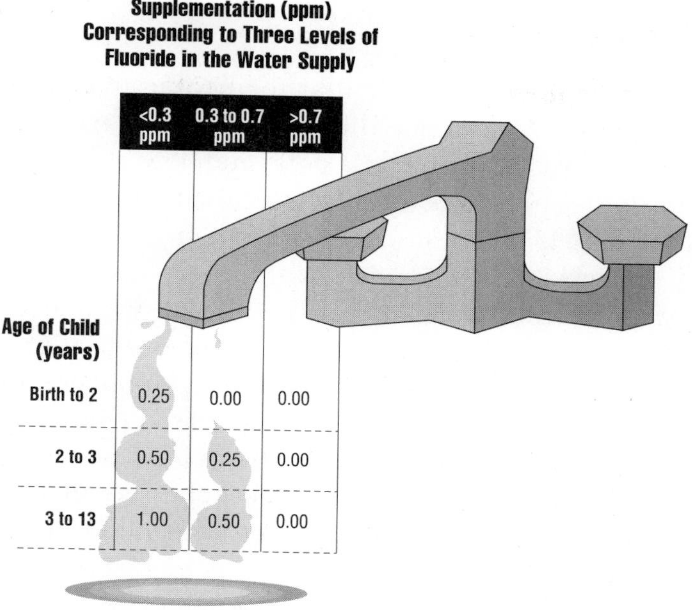

FIGURE 8.1 Recommended daily fluoride supplements for children in three age categories, based on fluoride concentration in the water supply. SOURCE: Recommendations by the Council on Dental Therapeutics of the American Dental Association, by the Committee on Nutrition of the American Academy of Pediatrics, and by the American Academy of Pediatric Dentistry.

lated to iron. It is also the most common and widespread nutritional disease in the world, though its overall prevalence in the United States is low compared with its prevalence in the rest of the world. Poor nutrition in infants and small children and blood loss and pregnancy in adults are the most frequent causes of iron deficiency. You might also be depriving yourself of iron if you do not eat many calories in the first place.

Women are particularly vulnerable to this cause of iron deficiency because they eat less food than men to begin with, but their requirements for iron are greater because they lose iron during menstruation. This may be one of the few cases where taking supplements is warranted, though you should do so only on the advice of your physician.

Potassium

The evidence is clear that for people with high blood pressure, potassium is one dietary factor that exerts a beneficial effect. This is partly because potassium lowers blood pressure and partly because it also protects against stroke and damage to blood vessels when blood pressure is high.

Several studies have shown that groups of people who eat low-potassium diets have an increased incidence of high blood pressure and heart disease. In addition, diets high in potassium and low in sodium can lower blood pressure. An intake of 3.5 g/day of potassium is associated with lower blood pressure and fewer deaths from strokes. All you have to do to get to this level of potassium is eat the five or more servings of fruit and vegetables a day recommended in the *Eat for Life* guidelines.

Sodium

Sodium is an essential nutrient, but the amount consumed by most people—mostly in the form of salt (sodium chloride)—well exceeds the amount needed for normal body function. Although the average adult needs no more than several hundred milligrams of sodium a day, surveys show that people consume between 4 and 5.8 g (4000 to 5800 mg) a day.

Although researchers have been studying the relationship of sodium to high blood pressure since the turn of the century, there is still some controversy about the importance of salt in regulating blood pressure. Many studies have shown, for example, that the higher a culture's average salt consumption, the higher the average blood pressure.

The controversy concerns what happens when individual people consume more or less salt—the effect on blood pressure varies tremendously. People differ greatly in their sensitivity to salt. In some, blood pressure is affected to a large extent by the amount of salt they eat. But other people can seemingly eat all the salt they want and not show any increase in blood pressure. Nevertheless, elevated blood pressure can develop very late in life.

Unfortunately, there is no easy way to measure salt sensitivity. Until there is, it makes sense for all of us to reduce our salt intake as a means of protecting ourselves against high blood pressure. If you already have high blood pressure, reducing the amount of sodium you eat may help lower your blood pressure.

A less important reason to restrict the amount of salt you eat is the increased incidence of stomach cancer in people who eat a great deal of salted, salt-cured, and pickled food. In countries where people eat a good deal of these foods, gastric cancer is relatively common. In Japan, the incidence of stomach cancer has declined in recent years as people are eating less salt-cured fish and salted vegetables. The incidence of stomach cancer is also declining in this country.

In food, sodium is present mainly in table salt. As a rule, 1 teaspoon of salt supplies 2000 mg of sodium. Some sodium in the diet comes from compounds such as sodium bicarbonate (baking soda), sodium citrate (a preservative), and monosodium glutamate (MSG, a flavor enhancer).

VITAMIN AND MINERAL SUPPLEMENTS

About 45 percent of the adult men and 55 percent of the adult women in the United States take a vitamin or mineral supplement either regularly or occasionally. Sales of dietary supplements have increased sixfold in the past 15 years, reaching $3 billion in 1987. The average U.S. adult who buys supplements spends about $32 a year for them.

People take supplements for a variety of reasons, most relating to a desire for better health and well-being. The odd thing is, people who take vitamin and mineral supplements tend to consume greater amounts of these nutrients in their foods than do people who do not take supplements. In other words, people who take supplements are more likely to meet their nutrient needs just from diet alone than people who do not take supplements—and who might actually need the extra nutrients.

The *Eat for Life* guidelines emphasize eating a balanced diet. By doing so, you will obtain all the vitamins and minerals you need to maximize your chances of staying in good health. Some vitamins and minerals are harmful in large doses, and people can get sick from overdosing on dietary supplements. Low levels of dietary supplements are safe, although they have not been shown to have any beneficial effect on health either. So unless your doctor specifically directs you to take a vitamin or mineral supplement for a specific medical reason, there is no reason for you to waste money on these preparations.

CHAPTER

9

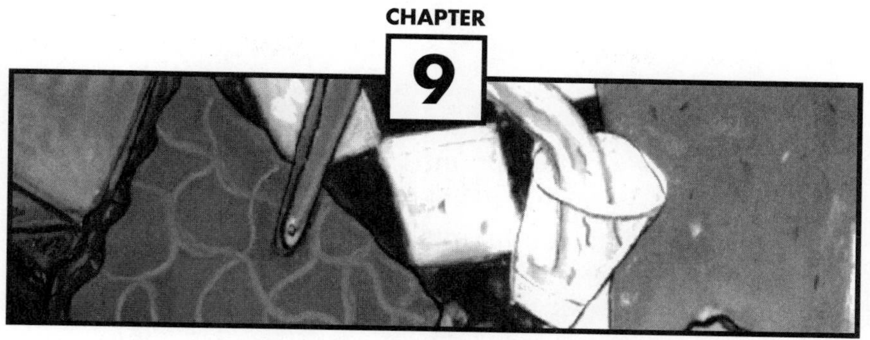

ALCOHOL, OTHER FOOD SUBSTANCES, AND CHRONIC DISEASES

The foods you eat and drink are more than just a combination of fats, carbohydrates, proteins, vitamins, and minerals. There are thousands of other substances present in food that also enter your body, some in minute quantities, others in large amounts. These food components do not serve any essential nutritional purpose, or at least none that we know about, and yet they might affect your body if you were to consume enough of them.

Ethanol, otherwise known as alcohol, is one example of a nonessential substance. Even though the body can use the 7 calories of energy provided by each gram of alcohol, it does not need alcohol to function—it can get the calories it needs from many food sources. In fact, there are no biochemical processes in the body that require alcohol. Caffeine—found in coffee, tea, and some soft drinks—and many of the trace chemicals that give food its flavor and smell are other examples of nonessential food substances that produce effects in the brain.

Food additives are another group of substances that you ingest almost daily. These include artificial colors and flavors, preservatives, and "texturizers," materials that give certain processed foods a desirable texture. Artificial sweeteners are another type of food additive.

There are also compounds in foods that are considered contaminants. This group of substances includes pesticide residues, environmental pollutants, and chemicals produced by microorganisms that might grow undetected on a food.

Evaluating the health effects of nonessential dietary substances is difficult. With alcohol, for example, it has been hard to determine with any accuracy how much people drink, mostly because people are reluctant to discuss their drinking habits with researchers. We consume such small amounts of most other nonessential substances that it is nearly impossible to detect any untoward effect on our health. So with those caveats in mind, here is what is known about the links between these substances and chronic diseases.

ALCOHOL

Alcohol, or actually beverages containing alcohol, has long been a part of human culture. Ancient Egyptians believed that *bouza*, what we call beer, was invented by the goddess Osiris and that it was both food and drink. Wine was also produced in ancient Egypt and was used in religious celebrations and as a medicine. Even then, wine was considered the aristocrat's drink, while beer was for the masses. In the New World, both the Aztec and the Incan societies valued alcoholic beverages made from fermented corn.

It was not until the first half of the eighteenth century that physicians in England recognized the adverse health consequences of alcohol. Soon afterward, the British Parliament passed the Gin Act of 1751, which made it more difficult and expensive to drink.

Figure 9.1 shows the alcohol content of beer, wine, and whiskey. There is no universally acceptable standard for the safe level of drinking, but for our purposes a light drinker is someone who downs between 0.01 and 0.21 ounces of alcohol a day—for example by having a bottle of beer or less every other day. A moderate drinker consumes between 0.22 and

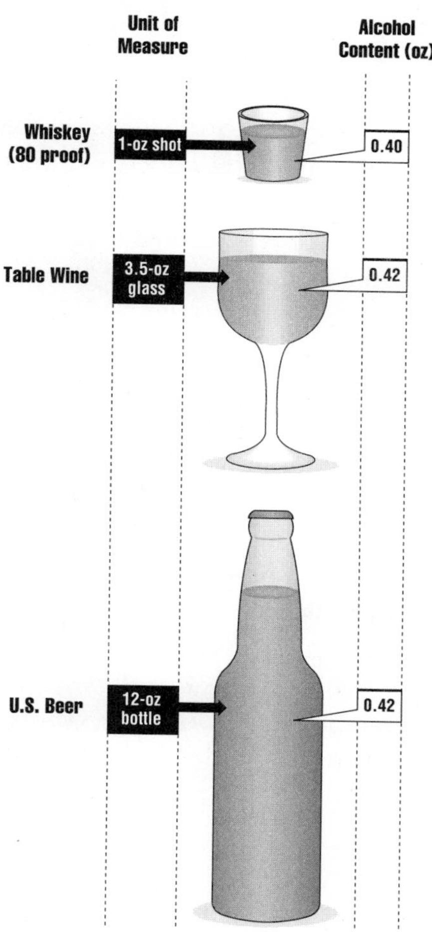

FIGURE 9.1 Amount of alcohol in a drink. Most table wines contain 11 to 13% alcohol. Fortified wines, such as sherry and port, contain approximately 20% alcohol. Most U.S. brands of beer contain 3.2 to 4.0% alcohol. SOURCE: Baum-Baicker, C. 1985. The health benefits of moderate alcohol consuption: a review of the literature. *Drug Alcohol Depend*. 15:207-227.

0.99 ounces of alcohol a day, perhaps by having a bottle of beer each day. Heavy drinkers consume an average of an ounce or more of alcohol each day. Nine percent of all adults in the United States are characterized as heavy drinkers, 24 percent are moderate drinkers, and 33 percent are light drinkers. The remaining 33 percent abstain from drinking.

The best indicator of the effect of drinking is the blood alcohol level. At a blood alcohol level of 0.05 (5 parts of alcohol to 10,000 parts of blood), which a person reaches after one or two drinks, most people experience positive sensations such as relaxation, euphoria, and well-being. Above this mark, a person starts feeling worse and gradually loses control of speech, balance, and emotions. When the blood alcohol level reaches 0.1, a person is drunk; at 0.2, some people pass out; at 0.3, some people collapse into a coma; and at 0.4 a person can die.

In 1985, some 18 million adults had problems with alcohol use. Of these, 41 percent, or 7.3 million adults, were alcohol abusers: they had experienced at least one moderately severe consequence of alcohol abuse, such as losing a job or being arrested, during the previous year. The remaining 59 percent, or 10.6 million adults, were alcoholics.

Alcohol abuse is more frequent in men than women and more common in youth and middle age. The *Eat for Life* guidelines do not recommend that you drink alcoholic beverages if you currently avoid them. But they do not recommend that you not use alcohol either (except during pregnancy), especially if you use it responsibly in limited amounts.

Liver Disease

Most cases of liver cirrhosis are caused by chronic heavy drinking. One study showed that drinking five drinks a day can cause cirrhosis in men. Women who drink heavily are more susceptible than men to cirrhosis; as few as three drinks a day can produce cirrhosis in women.

Although heavy drinking can lead to liver disease, only

about 18 percent of all alcoholics have cirrhosis. Perhaps this is because many alcoholics die from other causes before cirrhosis sets in. One study estimated that it takes an average of 25 years of drinking 7.5 ounces of alcohol—about one-third of a bottle of liquor—a day to produce cirrhosis. Compared with not drinking at all, downing 3.5 to 7 ounces of alcohol a day increases the risk of developing cirrhosis fivefold. Drinking even more than that makes it 25 times more likely that the drinker will develop cirrhosis.

Cancer

There is consistent evidence that alcohol increases the risk of cancers at several sites in the body, including the mouth, throat, esophagus, larynx, and liver. For cancer of the mouth, throat, esophagus, and larynx, drinking and smoking cigarettes appear to act synergistically to cause cancer. In other words, the damage caused by smoking and drinking together is worse than if you merely added the damage caused separately by each activity.

In North America and Western Europe, drinking is the main cause of cirrhosis of the liver, and cirrhosis is a primary cause of liver cancer. This does not mean, necessarily, that drinking causes liver cancer, though it does show that drinking produces a condition that may itself lead to liver cancer. However, some studies suggest that liver cancer may be more common in alcoholics even in the absence of cirrhosis, suggesting that alcohol itself may indeed cause liver cancer.

For women, heavy drinking may increase the risk of developing breast cancer. Several studies have found that among groups of women the incidence of breast cancer increases with the amount of alcohol consumed. But because some investigations have failed to find this association, the connection between alcohol consumption and breast cancer is far from proven.

Alcohol may cause cancer by a variety of mechanisms. Some experiments show, for example, that alcohol activates enzymes that can produce other cancer-causing chemicals within the body. Alcohol may also damage DNA, the gigantic molecule of which the body's genetic material is made. This, in turn, can cause a cell to begin multiplying uncontrollably.

Stroke and Heart Disease

People who regularly drink an average of two or more alcoholic beverages a day have higher average blood pressure levels and higher numbers of strokes than do people who are light drinkers or abstainers. In addition, heavy drinking increases the chances of suffering a stroke.

Heavy drinking is also associated with a greater chance of suffering a heart attack. On the other hand, moderate drinking may afford some protection against heart disease. A large study in Hawaii showed that men who are light or moderate drinkers have fewer heart attacks than men who either drink heavily or do not drink at all. In women, the "benefits" of drinking are not as apparent as they are in men.

Obesity

It is not unreasonable to think that alcohol may contribute to obesity, since for some people it can be a major calorie source. Drinking two beers a day would provide an additional 2100 calories a week. Over the course of several months, those extra calories might be expected to add a few inches to the waistline. And, indeed for some people, the extra calories from alcohol do translate into extra weight. But alcohol also increases the body's metabolic rate, causing it to burn calories at a higher rate than normal. Thus, although consuming alcohol may contribute too many calories to the diet, it is not the main cause of obesity.

Nervous System Diseases

Chronic drinking can damage the nervous system, producing dementia, confusion, difficulty in walking, and memory loss. It appears that thiamin deficiency, which results from heavy drinking, produces most of the damage to the nervous system. Alcohol does, however, also have direct toxic effects on brain cells.

Pregnancy

Women who drink heavily while pregnant can give birth to babies with fetal alcohol syndrome, which is characterized by a number of physical defects and behavioral disturbances. Less severe, though certainly noticeable, effects can also occur with even moderate drinking. Women who have as little as one drink a day during pregnancy are more likely than women who abstain from drinking while pregnant to deliver smaller babies. Thus the best advice if you are pregnant, or even thinking about getting pregnant, is not to drink.

COFFEE AND TEA

Tea's use as a beverage started in China in approximately 350 A.D. Coffee is a newer drink, first swallowed hot around 1000 A.D. Today, coffee and tea are among the most commonly consumed beverages in the world. In the United States, over half the adult population drinks coffee, with each person averaging 1.74 cups a day. Nearly 80 percent of the coffee is "regular," though the popularity of decaffeinated coffee is growing. Only about 31 percent of the U.S. population drinks tea. Coffee and tea are the greatest source of caffeine in the U.S. diet.

Cancer

There is no convincing evidence that drinking coffee or tea increases the chances of developing cancer. Some studies have suggested that coffee drinking might be associated with an increased risk of developing cancers of the bladder and colon, which prompted newspaper and magazine stories cautioning against coffee drinking. However, further investigations have exonerated coffee drinking; it appears that cigarette smoking was to blame for the increase in bladder cancer cases, and some other dietary factor, such as fats, may be at work with colon cancer.

Heart Disease

Over the past few years, a number of studies have found that coffee drinking may increase LDL-cholesterol levels, especially when the coffee is boiled (as it is in Scandinavia). But at least among U.S. coffee drinkers, the effect is so small as not to increase the risk for heart disease. Tea drinking has no effect on serum cholesterol levels, nor does it increase the risk of heart disease.

Pregnancy

In humans, caffeine crosses the placenta. In addition, the body metabolizes caffeine one-third as fast during pregnancy. As a result, caffeine accumulates in the mother, and it passes to the fetus, which has no enzymes with which to get rid of this chemical. What caffeine does to the human fetus is unclear, but some studies have shown that pregnant women who have high caffeine intakes are at greater risk of delivering babies of low birth weight. It appears sensible to limit caffeine intake during pregnancy.

OTHER FOOD ADDITIVES

Nearly 3,000 substances are added intentionally to foods in the United States during processing. Some 12,000 chemicals, such as the food packaging material polyvinyl chloride, can enter food more or less by accident; these are called indirect additives. However, the amount of most of these substances that we might eat during the course of a year is small. Here the safety records of a few of the most widely used additives are reviewed.

The most studied of all food additives is the artificial sweetener saccharin. Though saccharin causes bladder cancer in some species of animals raised in the laboratory, there is no convincing evidence of a link between saccharin and bladder cancer in humans.

Aspartame, another artificial sweetener, does not appear to cause cancer, either. And at levels 2 to 3 times higher than even the biggest diet soda drinkers would consume, aspartame does not produce any other harmful effects. However, people with the rare genetic disorder phenylketonuria should avoid foods flavored with aspartame, and these foods carry a warning label to this effect.

Nitrite is a common preservative in lunch meats and other cured meat products. It also occurs naturally in many foods and in human saliva. A recent survey found that the average U.S. diet contains approximately 0.8 mg of nitrite per day. More than one-third of the nitrite comes from cured meats; baked goods and cereals provide another third, and vegetables contribute about one-fifth of the nitrite in the U.S. diet. The nitrite in baked goods, cereals, and vegetables is there naturally, whereas the nitrite in cured meats is added as a preservative.

By itself, nitrite is probably not a cancer-causing substance. But nitrite can react with other naturally occurring chemicals to form nitrosamines, compounds that are carcinogenic. Smoke also contains significant levels of nitrosamines. Several studies in different parts of the world have shown that people who frequently eat cured pickles and meat and smoked foods have a higher risk of developing stomach cancer than people who eat such foods sparingly. One study showed that the odds of getting stomach cancer increased nearly threefold for every milligram of nitrite in the diet. It would be prudent therefore to limit the amount of smoked and cured foods that you eat, many of which are high in saturated fats anyway.

Two of the most common food additives are the preservatives BHA (butylated hydroxyanisole) and BHT (butylated hydroxytoluene). They are used extensively in dry cereals, shortenings, instant potato products, active dry yeast, and dry drink and dessert mixes. These two compounds have been around for many years, with no convincing evidence that they cause cancer or any other chronic diseases. There is no evidence, either, that the 100 or so milligrams of various food colors that we eat every day increases our risk of developing cancer.

Many of the indirect contaminants present in food can cause illness in humans at high levels. The amounts found in food, though, are so small that any risk they might pose is negligible. The one exception to this might be the microbial contaminant called aflatoxin, produced by a mold that infects corn and peanuts. Aflatoxin is among the most potent cancer-causing substances known, and its effect is mostly in the liver. In parts of Africa and Asia, it is not uncommon for people to eat corn and peanut products contaminated with aflatoxin. In those parts of the world, the incidence of liver cancer is much higher than anywhere else. In the United States an effort is made to limit the amount of aflatoxin that gets into the food supply, though we still consume minute amounts daily. Nevertheless, liver cancer is still a rare disease in this country.

Overall, there is not enough safety information on the complete range of nonnutritive additives and contaminants present in our food. But it seems unlikely that they contribute to our overall risk of chronic disease.

But just to play it safe, wash your fresh fruit and vegetables to remove traces of pesticides that might be present on the surface. And do not eat the seemingly unspoiled parts of moldy or spoiled foods, for although they appear okay, they may in fact contain microbial contaminants.

CHAPTER

10

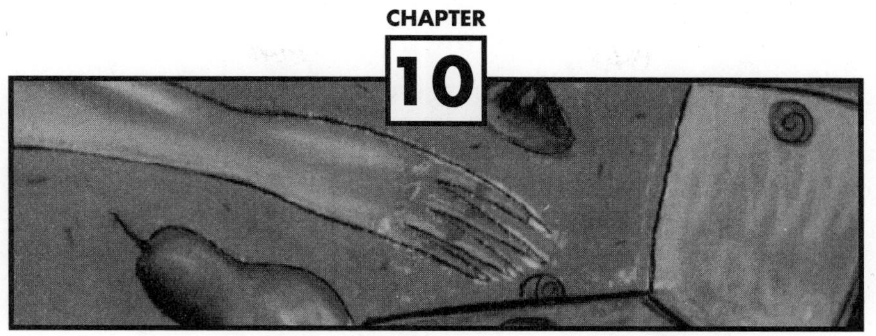

MAKING THE CHANGE TO THE NEW EATING PATTERN

After reading the first nine chapters of this book, you should be convinced that diet can play an important role in causing chronic diseases, including heart disease, cancers, high blood pressure, and stroke. It should also be clear that changing your diet can help to reduce your risk for these chronic diseases and therefore increase your chances of living a long and healthy life.

Now you must be wondering *how* to actually accomplish these changes. What types of food should you eat? What types of meals should you plan? Do you need to make changes in how you shop and cook? What can you eat at restaurants? In short, how do you translate the *Eat for Life* guidelines into a real, practical eating pattern?

WHAT FOODS SHOULD I EAT? SOME GENERAL GUIDELINES

Following the nine *Eat for Life* guidelines is mainly a matter of choosing the right foods to eat. Your main emphasis should be on limiting the amount of fat, saturated fatty acids, and cholesterol that you eat; eliminating added salt from your diet; eating more complex carbohydrates; eating a moderate amount of protein; and cutting down on your consumption of added sugars. In addition, you need to exercise enough to balance out the number of calories you consume.

You will need to select leaner cuts of meat, moving away from grades of meat that are heavily marbled with fat. Trim your meat of any excess chunks of fat, and remove the skin from poultry. And eat smaller and fewer portions of meat. Also, replace some of the meat you normally eat with fish and shellfish.

You should also get more of your protein from plant sources. Legumes—beans and peas—are good sources of both protein and complex carbohydrates. So, too, are cereal grains, such as whole wheat, rye, corn, and rice. So the next time you make chili, replace some of the ground beef with ground turkey and kidney beans. It will taste good but have significantly less fat, saturated fatty acids, and cholesterol.

Dairy products are an important source of calcium and protein, but whole milk, whole-milk cheeses and yogurt, ice cream, and other whole-milk products are high in saturated fatty acids. Therefore you need to emphasize low-fat and nonfat, or skimmed, milk products.

Since eggs yolks are high in cholesterol and saturated fatty acids, substitute an egg white for every other whole egg you use in a recipe. For example, if you normally eat a two-egg omelet, use one whole egg and one egg white, and add a little skim milk to the mixture.

Perhaps the simplest change to make is to switch from butter and lard to margarine with a low saturated fatty acid content. Margarine made from canola oil, for example, is rich in monounsaturated fatty acids, which when substituted for saturated fatty acids help lower LDL-cholesterol levels. Also, use less oil and fat in your cooking. Go easy on the salad dressing and limit fried foods in your diet.

Cutting down on fats in your diet means you will need to get more of your calories from carbohydrates. Eat more potatoes, bread, and whole-grain cereals, but go easy on bakery goods such as pies, pastries, and cookies since these are typically high in fat, saturated fatty acids, and added sugars.

Besides cutting out fat, limit your use of the salt shaker and sugar bowl at the table. Go easy on the salt, too, when cooking. If you now eat a lot of salt, your food may taste a little bland at first. Try other seasonings instead. You will be surprised at how good food tastes and how much better it gets as your taste buds adjust over the next few weeks.

Eat more fruits and vegetables. Though they contribute little in the way of calories, they are excellent sources of vitamins, minerals, and dietary fiber. They also add flavor to foods, making the transition to a reduced-salt diet even easier.

PLANNING A MENU

Sitting down with your family, a pile of cookbooks, and a list of favorite recipes in front of you and planning meals for the week ahead can be an enjoyable part of ensuring that your eating pattern is a healthful one. But besides being fun, planning your meals is an important part of eating to reduce your risk of chronic disease. For one thing, meal planning allows you to see in advance where the fat, cholesterol, and salt in your diet are coming from, information that can help you develop a more healthful eating pattern. If you know, for example, that you are going to have a hot dog and fries—a high-fat meal—at the ballpark Wednesday night, then you might choose dishes that are particularly low in fat and cholesterol for the meals before and after. You need to be concerned only with the average nutritional content of your diet, not every single food and every single meal. Meal planning offers other benefits, such as saving time and money. Shopping for specific foods for several days of meals takes less time than shopping haphazardly or for just one day at a time. In addition, shopping for these foods, a topic covered later in this chapter, will reduce the amount of food—and therefore money—that goes to waste in your refrigerator because you forgot to use it.

Planning meals should also help keep you from getting into an eating rut. Each time you sit down to plan your meals, bring out the family recipe file and your cookbooks and look for favorite meals that you may have neglected for some time. Keep an eye out, too, for new recipes in newspapers and magazines. While some of these will probably be high in fat, cholesterol, and salt, it is not difficult to modify most recipes so that they are easier to fit into a dietary pattern that meets the *Eat for Life* guidelines without losing their appeal, as you will learn in the section on cooking below.

There are three keys to planning an eating pattern that is delicious and nutritious and that helps to reduce your risk of chronic disease. The first is to meet the recommendations for daily servings of fruits and vegetables and complex carbohydrates. Filling your menu each day with at least five servings a day of fruits and vegetables and six servings of cereals, breads, and legumes will give you many of the vitamins and minerals you need without adding fat, saturated fatty acids, cholesterol, and salt to your diet. This is assuming, of course, that your complex carbohydrates do not come from French fries, potato chips, and donuts and that you do not cover your vegetables with lots of fatty salad dressings.

The second key is to develop a feel for which foods are low in fats, saturated fatty acids, cholesterol, and salt, and which are not. In some foods, you can see the fat and salt, while in others it is hidden. The visible fats are easy to spot—the marbling in meat, oil in salad dressings, butter on bread, cream bases for soups and sauces. Examples of hidden fats are the butterfat in whole milk and cheese, cooking oil absorbed by French fries, the fat in many cookies and crackers, and the oil in avocados and nuts. You can often see the salt on foods like pretzels, peanuts, and crackers, but salt is also added to many processed foods and is a component of steak and soy sauces.

There are some foods that you might think are high in fat but really are not. Pizza, for example, easily fits into a moderate-fat diet. Two slices of a typical 12-inch cheese pizza contain only about 350 calories, of which only about 16 percent are fat, and 10 milligrams (mg) of cholesterol. Topping it with onions, green peppers, and mushrooms adds a few calories, but no fat. Those two slices also supply a good amount of calcium and iron. The only drawback to pizza is that it contains about 1.5 g of salt, one-quarter of the daily maximum. For those foods for which you have no clue as to their fat content, consult the references recommended in Appendix B.

The third key to healthful eating is to limit the amount of meat, poultry, and seafood that you eat. You do not have to eliminate these foods entirely from your diet, but try to eat smaller portions—about 3 ounces per meal, with a maximum of 6 ounces per day, is a good compromise. Trim any visible fat from the meat and poultry and buy lean cuts. (For more advice, see the sections later in this chapter on shopping for meat, poultry, and seafood.)

In planning your eating pattern, you do not have to ignore snacks and desserts. A wisely chosen snack can add an extra serving of complex carbohydrates or fruit to your daily intake. Fruit is an excellent snack. So is air-popped popcorn; it's filling and virtually all complex carbohydrates. Limit snacks that are high in fat, added sugar, and salt, the main nutritional disadvantages for most snack foods sold in the United States. In small amounts, some crackers are good snacks, although some are high in saturated fatty acids. If you love pretzels, look for low-salt or no-salt varieties.

Desserts need not be fat-filled creations, either. Angel food cake, for example, is virtually fat-free. Desserts centered on fruits are your best bet for low-fat dishes without much added sugar. Fruit cobblers, crisps, and compotes are good choices. But even cookies and ice cream, though high in fat, occasionally can be a part of your diet. Just don't eat large quantities of them.

Menu planning may seem time-consuming now, but with practice you will find that it becomes much easier. For example, chances are good that when you sit down to plan your meals, you will think of more meals than you can eat in a week. Jot those down for the following week.

SHOPPING

Now that you know what you are going to eat, you will need to make a trip to the grocery store. To become a smart shopper, you must learn how to read food labels, how to look for lean meats, and how to read past some of the "health" claims on product labels in order to get to the real nutritional content of an item. The following sections will help you to develop these skills.

Fruits and Vegetables

Perhaps the single best place to start shopping is the produce department. Here there is little fat, salt, added sugar, or cholesterol. The two exceptions are avocados and coconuts. Because both are high in fat (coconuts in particular are rich in saturated fatty acids), you should eat them in moderation at best.

The produce aisle is a good place to find new foods to enliven your diet. In the lettuce section, for example, try leaf, bibb, Boston, or romaine lettuce or endive. Use fresh spinach to add variety—and nutrients—to your salad bowl. If you like spicy foods, use a small amount of hot-tasting mustard greens in your tossed salad.

Potatoes are a great source of complex carbohydrates and some vitamins and minerals. So, too, are sweet potatoes, which you can bake just like regular white potatoes. Squashes are poorly appreciated by most U.S. adults, but they are simple to cook and cheap and plentiful in winter when many vegetables go up in cost. Next time you make boiled potatoes, add a turnip or parsnip to the pot as well.

Many fruits are good sources of vitamins and minerals. For example, bananas are one of the best sources of potassium. Citrus fruits are the best natural source of vitamin C, and watermelon supplies a good bit of vitamin C and carotenoids for vitamin A.

Grain Products

Grain products include breads and cereals made from wheat, rye, corn, rice, and other grains. They are rich in complex carbohydrates and usually low in fat. The notable fatty exceptions are croissants, pastries, cakes, and granola. By combining grain products with meat, poultry, or fish, you will reduce your dependence on these animal foods as the centerpiece of dinner. Try combining rice or pasta, for example, with lightly sautéed vegetables, beans, and herbs and spices—perhaps with a small amount of beef, chicken, or fish—to make a nutritious, low-fat entrée.

Eat plenty of grain products each day, but try to select those made with whole or unrefined grains as often as possible. Foods like whole wheat bread, brown rice, oatmeal, and cereal and pasta made from whole grains are not as heavily refined as white bread, white rice, and corn flakes, for example, so they have more vitamins, minerals, and fiber.

Legumes

Most people should eat more legumes (or beans, as they are more commonly called). Black beans, pinto beans, kidney beans, navy beans, soybeans, black-eyed peas, split green or yellow peas, chick peas (garbanzos), and lentils contain plenty of complex carbohydrates, fiber, protein, vitamins, and minerals. They are also inexpensive and low in fat. One cup of cooked kidney beans, for example, contains less than 1 g of fat.

Legumes are versatile foods. Add them to salads, for example, or to dishes where meat or cheese are combined with a grain and vegetables. Substitute lentils for some or all of the ground beef when making meat sauce for spaghetti.

Legumes like lentils or split peas can be prepared in under an hour, but you have to boil others for several hours to make them edible. You can buy many legumes in cans or frozen packages, ready to use. Drain or rinse them before use to remove the salt or sugar in the packaging liquid. Beware of canned refried beans, however, which can be high in fat.

Dairy Products

As a group, dairy products are the best sources of calcium in the U.S. diet, but they are also the second-largest source of saturated fatty acids. Food manufacturers are now making cheeses and other dairy products that have less fat and salt than those we are used to eating. For example, while part-skim-milk mozzarella cheese has been available for years, you can now find part-skim Swiss, muenster, jack, cheddar, and cream cheeses as well as skim-milk ricotta cheese. Some of these new products have less than half the fat and cholesterol of their whole-milk cousins. Many of them are lower in sodium as well.

Regular large-curd cottage cheese seems to be a good buy because the package says it is only 4 percent fat. But that only means that fat constitutes 4 percent of the total weight of the product. In fact, 40 percent of the calories in regular cottage cheese comes from fat. Low-fat cottage cheeses, in contrast, get 13 to 18 percent of their calories from fat. Dry curd cottage cheese, which is crumbly, gets only 7 percent of its calories from fat.

When buying milk, choose skim milk or 1 percent milk. Two percent milk is not as low fat as you might think; although it is 2 percent fat by weight, it actually gets 36 percent of its calories from fat. Whole milk, in contrast, derives almost half its calories from fat. Most buttermilk is made from skim or 1 percent milk.

Yogurts, too, come in several forms. One 8-ounce carton of regular yogurt, made from whole milk, contains 140 calories, half of which comes from fat. A carton of low-fat yogurt, made from partially skimmed milk, contains 113 calories, of which 30 percent comes from fat. Nonfat yogurt, made from skim milk, is virtually fat free; one carton contains about 90 calories.

One myth about margarine is that it is less fattening than butter. In fact, butter and margarine contain the same amount of calories per serving—all of it from fat. However, margarine has no cholesterol and less saturated fatty acids than butter. Don't be deceived by the "no cholesterol" claims of some margarines, for all margarines are cholesterol-free—they are made from cholesterol-free vegetable oils.

Brands of margarine do differ, however, in the amount and types of saturated fatty acids they contain, and most margarine packages list the number of grams of saturated and polyunsaturated fatty acids in one serving. Buy brands that are lowest in saturated fatty acids.

Meats and Poultry

Meats constitute the biggest source of fat in the U.S. diet. Limiting the amount of meat in your meals is one way to reduce your fat intake. Other ways include picking lower-fat cuts of meat and eating meat less often.

When buying meat, whether it is beef, pork, or poultry, purchase just enough to provide about 4 ounces per serving uncooked, which will yield 3-ounce servings when cooked. The meat from one chicken leg and a thigh, or a half chicken breast, weighs about 4 ounces uncooked. So does a piece of beef or pork about the size of a deck of cards.

Chicken and turkey, minus the skin, are low in fat, saturated fatty acids, and cholesterol. White meat has less fat than dark meat. Duck and goose, however, are high in fat, so do not make them part of your regular diet.

Choosing beef is a little more complicated, since different parts of the cow naturally contain different amounts of fat. In addition, some cows are fattier than others. One clue to the fat content of a piece of meat is its grade. Prime beef, because it is heavily marbled, is the highest in fat content, followed by choice and select. Some grocery stores give a special "lean" designation to select-grade cuts that are trimmed of most visible fat. All four grades contain about the same amount of cholesterol, though, because cholesterol is found mainly in the muscle itself as opposed to the fat. Choice cuts of beef can contain about one-third less fat than prime cuts; the fat content of select cuts is only about one-half that of prime beef.

Fat content differs, too, according to the specific cut of beef. This is true of pork as well. Table 10.1 is a list of cuts of beef, pork, and poultry to buy that will help you reduce the amount of fat in your diet. Try to pick the select or choice grades, but regardless of which cuts of meat you choose, trim all the visible fat before you cook it.

Seafood

Fish is a delicious, low-fat source of protein that could easily replace some of the beef and pork you probably now

TABLE 10.1 Choosing Meats to Reduce Fat and Cholesterol

Name of Cut	Calories	Fat (grams)	Saturated Fatty Acids (grams)	Cholesterol (milligrams)
Beef (lean only, choice grade)				
Top round steak, broiled	160	5	2	70
Eye of round, roasted	150	5	2	60
Tip round, roasted	150	5	2	70
Sirloin, broiled	170	7	3	75
Top loin, broiled	180	8	3	65
Tenderloin, broiled	180	9	3	70
Bottom round, braised	180	7	3	80
Chuck arm pot roast, braised	190	7	3	85
Pork (lean only)				
Tenderloin, roasted	140	4	1	70
Ham, boneless, water added, extra lean (approximately 5% fat)	110	4	1	40
Ham, roasted	125	5	2	45
Center loin chop, broiled	170	7	3	70
Poultry (roasted)				
Turkey light meat, without skin	130	3	1	60
Chicken breast, meat only	140	3	1	70
Chicken drumstick, meat only	145	5	1	80
Chicken breast, meat and skin	170	7	2	70
Chicken drumstick, meat and skin	185	9	3	75

NOTE: These meats are generally good choices when you are limiting fat and cholesterol in your diet. All the figures shown are for 3-ounce servings with all visible fat removed. None of the meats was prepared with added fat.

Eating up to two 3-ounce servings of these meats, along with other low-fat, low-cholesterol food choices, allows you to limit the amount of fat you eat to less than 30 percent of your total calories and limit cholesterol to less than 300 milligrams daily.

SOURCE: U.S. Department of Agriculture, Human Nutrition Information Service.

eat. Even the fattiest fishes have only about as much fat as the leanest meats. More importantly, fish fat is low in saturated fatty acids and high in unsaturated fatty acids, particularly those of the omega-3 family (see Chapter 3).

Fish and shellfish are comparable to lean meat and poultry in cholesterol content, but supply less saturated and total fat. Only shrimp, with about 165 mg of cholesterol in a 3-ounce serving, has more cholesterol than lean meat, although, again, it has less fat than beef, pork, or poultry.

Vegetable Oils

They may look the same, but all cooking oils are not alike. For one thing, several of them have a discernible flavor—olive oil and peanut oil, for example. They also differ in their fat composition—the types of fats they contain. Figure 10.1 shows some of the common cooking oils as well as butter, lard, and beef fat for comparison.

As you can see, canola oil is the lowest in saturated fatty acids, whereas coconut oil is the highest. Canola oil is also rich in monounsaturated fatty acids, as is olive oil. Both oils are good to use in cooking.

Packaged Meats

Like the dairy case, the packaged meat refrigerator containing bacon, sausage, and lunch meats has begun to slim down. Bacon and sausage are still high in fat, cholesterol, and salt, and it is best to limit your purchases of those foods. Some lunch meats, however, are losing some of their fat. Turkey cold cuts, for example, can have less than 1 g or as much as 5 g of fat per slice. Still, at 1 or 2 g of fat per slice, a sandwich with two slices of meat, lettuce, and tomato will make it easy for you to have a lowfat lunch.

Be careful of potentially misleading claims that appear, for example, on hot dog packages, which say that

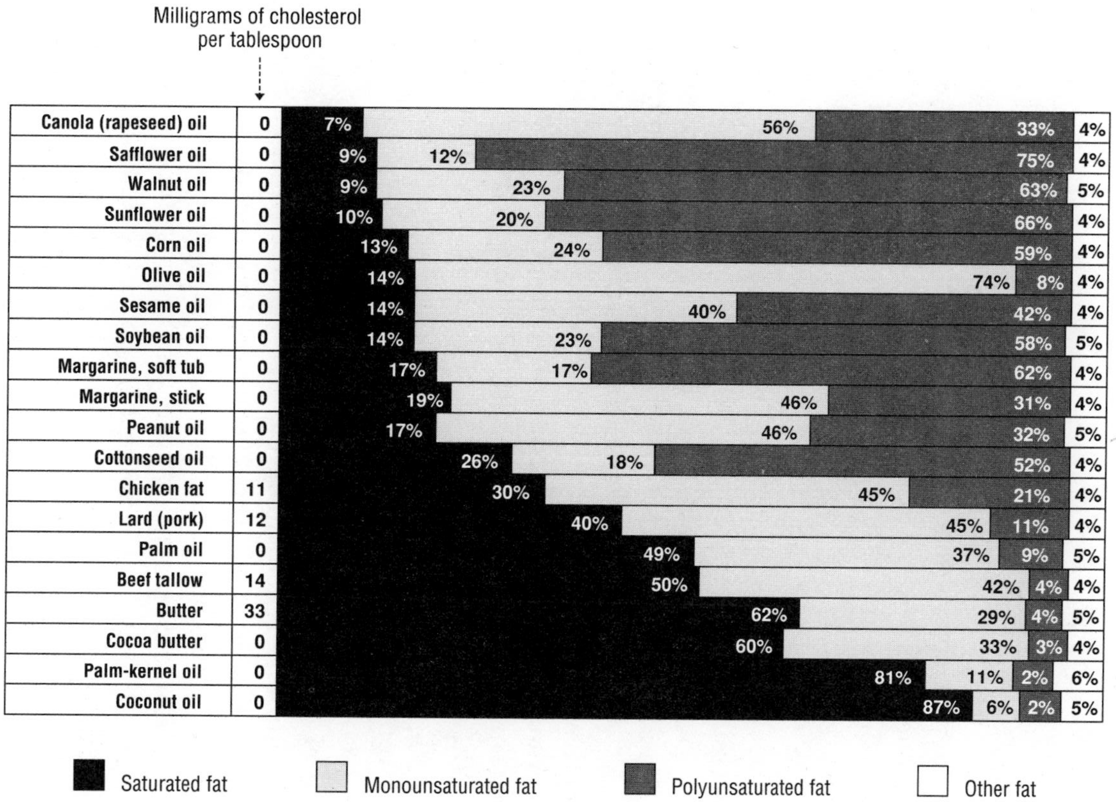

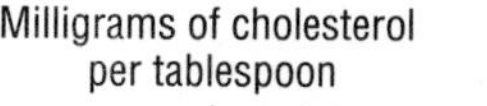

	Milligrams of cholesterol per tablespoon	Saturated fat	Monounsaturated fat	Polyunsaturated fat	Other fat
Canola (rapeseed) oil	0	7%	56%	33%	4%
Safflower oil	0	9%	12%	75%	4%
Walnut oil	0	9%	23%	63%	5%
Sunflower oil	0	10%	20%	66%	4%
Corn oil	0	13%	24%	59%	4%
Olive oil	0	14%	74%	8%	4%
Sesame oil	0	14%	40%	42%	4%
Soybean oil	0	14%	23%	58%	5%
Margarine, soft tub	0	17%	17%	62%	4%
Margarine, stick	0	19%	46%	31%	4%
Peanut oil	0	17%	46%	32%	5%
Cottonseed oil	0	26%	18%	52%	4%
Chicken fat	11	30%	45%	21%	4%
Lard (pork)	12	40%	45%	11%	4%
Palm oil	0	49%	37%	9%	5%
Beef tallow	14	50%	42%	4%	4%
Butter	33	62%	29%	4%	5%
Cocoa butter	0	60%	33%	3%	4%
Palm-kernel oil	0	81%	11%	2%	6%
Coconut oil	0	87%	6%	2%	5%

FIGURE 10.1 Here's how the fats compare. Each of these fats has been analyzed to show the proportions of saturated, monounsaturated, and polyunsaturated fatty acids. Limit those fats that contain a higher proportion of saturated fatty acids. Notice that some fats contain no cholesterol but have large proportions of saturated fatty acids. SOURCE: *Mayo Clinic Nutrition Letter* with permission of Mayo Foundation for Medical Education and Research, Rochester, MN 55905.

franks contain no more than 30 percent fat. All hot dogs, by law, contain no more than 30 percent fat—by weight. But by calories, hot dogs and other sausage products are about 80 percent fat.

Packaged Goods

When it comes to buying foods that are enclosed in boxes or packages (including many of those discussed above), the key to being a smart shopper is to read the label carefully. Look past the claims that an item is "low-fat" or "lite." What is "lite" in the eyes of the manufacturer may really be laden with fat. Salad dressings are a good example: some "lite" salad dressings get nearly 80 percent of their calories from fat. Look for brands that contain 1 g or less of fat per tablespoon.

Similarly, soups and spaghetti sauces are likely to make "low salt" claims. One spaghetti sauce may be "low salt" compared with another, but even the less salty brand most likely contains substantial amounts of salt. Look for brands that contain no added salt or are very low in sodium.

When selecting packaged goods, check the ingredient list carefully. By law, the ingredients are listed in order by weight, from greatest to least. Sometimes, to disguise a highly sweetened product, for example, manufacturers will use a combination of sweeteners so that the word "sugar" does not appear high up on the list of ingredients. Here is a list of common sugar replacements: corn sweeteners, corn syrup, dextrose, fructose, fruit juice concentrate, high fructose corn syrup, honey, invert sugar, maltose, maple syrup, and molasses.

Directly above the ingredient list on most packaged goods is the nutritional information. Figure 10.2 shows the nutritional information from a 15-ounce box of soda crackers. The information here is straightforward. Eating 10 crackers provides 120 calories: 12 calories from protein (3 g times 4 calories per gram of protein), 80 calories from carbohydrates (20 g times 4 calories per gram of carbohydrate), and 36 calories from fat (4 g times 9 calories per gram of fat.) You will notice that 12 + 80 + 36 = 128, not 120. In this case, the manufacturers are not trying to deceive you; they round off the amount of protein, carbohydrates, and fat to the nearest gram to avoid using decimal points on the label. Even with rounding, you can determine that fat accounts for roughly 30 percent of the calories (36 divided by 120 times 100 percent) in the crackers.

Keep in mind that the serving size on the label may have nothing to do with the way you really eat. For example, do you usually eat 10 crackers with a bowl of soup? If not,

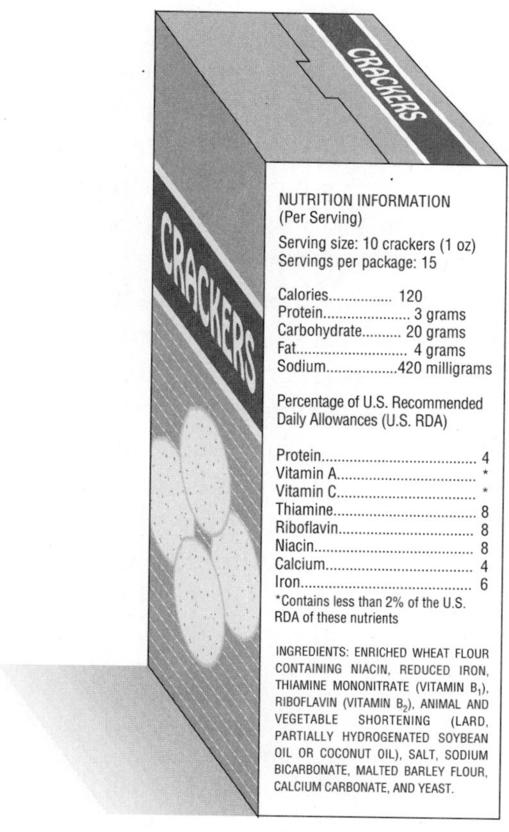

FIGURE 10.2 Nutritional information from a box of soda crackers.

you have to figure out how much fat you are getting from the number of crackers you do eat.

Unfortunately, most food labels do not yet provide information on the kind of fat the product contains. However, you can get some clues by looking at the list of ingredients. Look for the types of shortening and vegetable oil in the product. Most crackers contain shortening. These crackers are made with lard plus either partially hydrogenated soybean oil or partially hydrogenated coconut oil. Lard, being an animal fat, is high in saturated fatty acids, particularly those fatty acids that raise LDL-cholesterol (see Chapter 3). Partially hydrogenated coconut oil is also high. Partially hydrogenated soybean oil, while not as high in saturated fatty acids as the other two, still contains a good deal of these cholesterol-raising fatty acids. It is safe to assume, then, that much of the fat in these crackers is LDL-cholesterol-raising saturated fatty acids. Crackers made with vegetable shortening alone are a better choice, especially if the shortening is partially hydrogenated soybean oil.

The information on vitamins and minerals in the middle of the label is clear. Foods that contain more than 10 percent of the U.S. RDA per serving are considered good sources of that nutrient. (U.S. RDAs are a set of values developed by the Food and Drug Administration to be used as standards for the nutritional labeling of foods and dietary supplements. See Appendix A.)

Not all packaged foods are labeled, though, because nutritional labeling is voluntary. The Food and Drug Administration is considering ways to improve the nutritional information on labels and to make labeling mandatory. Until new regulations go into effect, you will have to make do with the labels now available.

Frozen Food

Reading labels carefully is a must in the frozen food section. For example, some frozen yogurts and tofu creations are low in fat, but others have as much or even more fat than ice cream. Also be careful with frozen entrees and TV dinners. Many of these are billed as "diet" foods. They may, indeed, be low in calories, but some are also high in fat, cholesterol, and salt. If you buy these products, choose wisely.

Frozen vegetables can be a good buy, particularly when the fresh vegetable is out of season. But products that come packed in butter or cream sauces can be high in saturated fatty acids, cholesterol, and salt.

COOKING

You have planned your menu wisely, and you have been a smart shopper. Now it's time to be a clever chef and prepare your meals with a minimum of fat and salt.

Methods and Equipment

Certain ways of cooking food are inherently better than others from a nutrition point of view. Steaming, for example, adds no fat to food and should become an important part of your cooking procedures. Deep-fat frying, on the other hand, adds loads of fat, and you should cook as little food as possible by this method.

Steaming vegetables—instead of boiling them—is a wonderful way to cook because it spares nutrients and keeps the vegetables tender. To steam vegetables, cut them into serving-size pieces and place them in the steamer basket. Put a half-inch or so of water in the bottom of the pot, nestle the basket inside, cover tightly, and turn on the heat. When steam starts escaping from the pot, turn the heat down and continue cooking. Do not remove the lid. Most vegetables will cook in 3 to 5 minutes. Some, such as Brussels sprouts, can take as much as 10 minutes, and artichokes require about 45 minutes.

The Chinese invented a good method for cooking with little fat called stir-frying, which uses intense heat and a small amount of oil to quick-cook vegetables and meat, sealing in flavor and nutrients. There are two keys to stir-frying: cutting the meat and vegetables into thin pieces and getting the pan hot and keeping it hot while you cook. The best pan for this is a wok, but a large cast-iron skillet will also work.

To cook in a wok, heat the pan over high heat and add a tablespoon or so of oil. Add whatever meat you are using, stirring until it is browned on all sides, which should take only a minute or two. Add slow-cooking vegetables such as broccoli and carrots first, stir for a minute or so, and then add quick-cooking vegetables such as green beans, snap peas, and bean sprouts. If the food begins to stick to the pan, add a little water, low-sodium broth, or salt-reduced soy sauce.

Sautéing is a common food preparation method that should be modified somewhat. Most recipes call for too much oil for sautéing; you can usually reduce the oil substantially, especially if you use a nonstick frying pan.

Broiling is a useful technique for sealing flavor into meats, poultry, and fish. Do not preheat the broiler, for then you are really baking food at high temperature. For the same reason, leave the broiler or oven door open slightly when broiling.

Beforehand, season food with herbs and spices, or soak it for several hours in a marinade.

Many people do not buy fish because they are not sure how to cook it. To cook fish under the broiler—or by any method—use the rule of ten: measure the piece of fish at its thickest point, and cook 10 minutes for every inch of thickness. In other words, a half-inch-thick fillet needs 5 minutes to cook; a one-inch-thick fish steak needs 10 minutes.

A microwave oven can save both calories and time. Fish and vegetables stay tender and fresh when cooked in a microwave with no added fat. Having a microwave also enables you to make quick, nutritious meals from frozen soups, pasta sauces, and some casseroles. This might keep you from visiting your favorite fast-food restaurant—and eating high-fat foods—when you do not have time to prepare a meal from scratch.

Substitutions

Many recipes in cookbooks or magazines were created for the age when we were ignorant about the effects of fat, cholesterol, and salt on our health. Unfortunately, many chefs and cookbook writers still choose to ignore what we know about diet and health, but that does not mean you have to. You can modify certain ingredients without changing the recipe significantly.

Eggs. The major source of cholesterol in the U.S. diet is the egg. One large egg yolk contains approximately 215 mg of cholesterol and nearly 5 g of fat, about 2 g of which is saturated.

Eggs play two roles in cooking. The yolks, because they are almost exclusively fat, add tenderness, smoothness, and richness to baked goods. The egg whites, which are mostly protein, provide structural strength.

In recipes that include margarine, shortening, or vegetable oil, simply use the egg white alone wherever a whole egg is called for. If you find that the resulting product is a little tough, next time add an extra teaspoon of vegetable oil along with the egg white. About the only time this substitution does not work is with pound cake or flourless cakes.

If the egg yolk is the only source of fat in the recipe, substitute one egg white and 1 teaspoon of vegetable oil. You can use the same substitution in recipes that use egg as a coating for meat.

If you love scrambled eggs or omelets, you have two options for reducing their fat and cholesterol content. Instead of using two whole eggs, use one egg and one egg white, and add a pinch of dried dillweed or chives to the eggs. The alternative is to use one of the egg substitute products available in the dairy case.

Egg whites themselves can be used to lower the amount of fat in certain baked goods. Next time you make a fruit pie, leave off the top crust and use a meringue—made from egg whites, cream of tartar, and sugar—instead. Meringue is also a good substitute for whipped cream as a dessert topping. Baked meringues, with a little almond or vanilla extract added, can replace cookies for dessert.

Dairy products. One easy change to make in the way you cook is to replace the whole milk in recipes with skim milk. In most cases, you can simply substitute skim milk for whole milk without making any other adjustments.

Nondairy coffee whiteners are poor substitutes for milk or cream; they are usually high in fat, often saturated fat. Instead, use a little skim milk and nonfat milk powder.

Cream soups will be a little thin using skim milk for whole milk or cream. Instead, use evaporated canned skim milk. Another option is to peel and slice thinly one potato, cook it in a little bit of water or in the microwave, and puree it with regular skim milk. The starch from the potato will thicken your soup enough that you will not notice the missing whole milk or cream.

Nonfat plain yogurt is a good substitute for sour cream in baked goods. When you make mashed potatoes, instead of adding butter and whole milk, use a tablespoon of yogurt and a splash of skim milk.

Yogurt cheese—made simply by draining off the liquid from nonfat plain yogurt in a cheesecloth-lined colander overnight and refrigerating for a day—is a good no-fat, no-cholesterol substitute for cream cheese in any recipe. It tastes and feels so much like cream cheese that you can even use it on toast.

Salad dressings. Use salad dressings sparingly. Most of them are high in fat and salt, but there are some available that are oil-free and low in sodium.

Condensed creamed soups. Instead of one can of condensed creamed soup, use a homemade white sauce with flavoring. To make a white sauce, melt 1 tablespoon of margarine in a saucepan. Stir in 2 tablespoons of flour, and cook over medium heat for a minute or two. Increase heat and slowly add 1 cup of skim milk while stirring. Cook until the sauce thickens.

To replace a can of cream of celery soup, add some finely chopped celery to your white sauce. For a can of mushroom soup, add finely chopped fresh mushrooms.

Salt. There is no doubt that salt can add to the flavor of food. But once you wean yourself from putting salt on everything you eat, you will be surprised at how good food tastes on its own and how salty most processed food tastes.

To help kick the salt habit, season your food with herbs and spices. The secret is to use these flavoring ingredients in moderation. Also, when experimenting with herbs and spices, do not use too many at once. Used sparingly, they add to the natural flavor of food rather than overwhelming it.

Sprinkling a little dried or fresh basil, tarragon, or dill on your salad, together with a squeeze of lemon, can add flavor to your favorite greens without adding calorie-laden salad dressing. When cooking chicken, add a sprig of rosemary or a pinch of tarragon to the dish. Lean hamburgers go well with a sprinkling of minced marjoram and chives and a slice of tomato.

Add a pinch of cayenne pepper or a dash of hot sauce to stews, soups, and casseroles. (By the way, recent studies have shown that spicy food does not irritate the stomach.) Commercially prepared spice and herb mixtures that contain little or no salt can promote flavorful low-salt cooking.

Meat. In recipes such as chili, meat sauce, or shepherd's pie that call for ground beef, you can substitute ground turkey; about 45 percent of the calories in ground turkey come from fat, whereas even the leanest ground beef gets about 50 percent of its calories from fat. The texture of cooked ground turkey is no different from that of ground beef, and in heavily seasoned dishes you will not be able to detect any difference in flavor, either.

EATING OUT

Food served in many restaurants and cafeterias in the United States tends to be high in fat, cholesterol, salt, and added sugar. Some changes are being made as chefs realize that consumers want and enjoy nutritious meals, but this shift is only beginning. Until it becomes more widespread, there are some things you can do to protect your health while enjoying a meal out.

The first thing you should know is that most chefs are eager to please the customer. The restaurant business is very competitive, and regular customers can make the difference between a restaurant's success or failure. An accommodating chef will often prepare dishes to order for you. If the fish listed on the menu is sautéd in butter, ask to have yours broiled with a little lemon. Sometimes your request can be as simple as putting sauces or dressings on the side. Most restaurants will also give you smaller servings if you request them. In many Chinese restaurants, each dish is prepared fresh, so you can ask that yours be prepared with only a small amount of salt.

In many cases, though, you can get a nutritious meal simply by choosing wisely from the menu. Some menus have special "healthy heart" selections—these are prepared to keep fat and salt content low. The so-called "diet plates," however, are no nutritional bargain. Usually, they consist of a hamburger minus the bun or mayonnaise-heavy tuna salad on a piece of lettuce—meals with very little carbohydrate but plenty of fat and protein. Look for foods that are baked, grilled, or broiled with lemon juice or wine instead of butter. Dishes prepared by steaming, roasting, or poaching also tend to be low in fat. By the same token, limit or avoid foods that are au gratin, buttered, creamy, marinated in oil, or fried. Cream, hollandaise, béchamel, cheese, and butter sauces are all fat heavy. Some chefs, influenced by French nouvelle cuisine, are using lighter sauces, but often these are lighter only because they do not use flour—they still use cream and butter. Also, watch out for smoked and pickled foods, or those served au jus, for they are likely to be salty.

Italian restaurants tend to be good choices for those in search of low-fat food. Eat only small portions of cheese- and meat-stuffed dishes, such as lasagna, ravioli, and manicotti, or split a stuffed dish with someone who orders pasta with red clam sauce. Marinara and marsala sauces are also low in fat. Chicken and fish cooked Italian style are often simply prepared using wine and herbs and thus are good selections.

Asian cuisines are usually low in fat and cholesterol because they rely heavily on vegetables and stir-frying. But be careful of fried appetizers like wontons and egg rolls, and dishes cooked in coconut milk. Szechuan dishes sometimes involve frying meat in hot oil. Remember, moderation is the key with foods such as these.

Pancakes are a good choice for a restaurant breakfast, but ask to have the butter served on the side, and leave most of it there. Order your toast, English muffin, or bagel plain, and use jam on it instead of butter: you get some added sugar, but no extra fat or cholesterol. Also, if you have an occasional egg, order it poached or soft-boiled instead of fried.

An increasing number of restaurants and cafeterias now offer salad bars with a wide range of selections. A well-stocked salad bar can provide a nutritious, low-fat meal if you choose vegetables, fruit, garbanzo beans, or flaked tuna or chicken. Cottage cheese, hard cheese, pasta salad, potato salad, guacamole, diced ham, and olives are okay, but only in small amounts; the ham and olives are salty, and the rest of these items are high in fat. Use little, if any, bacon bits, chopped eggs, pickled foods, and regular salad dressings. If you want dressing, choose a low-calorie selection or use lemon and a sprinkling of pepper with perhaps a bit of oil.

Fast food is often rich in fat, cholesterol, and salt, but this situation is changing. Fast-food restaurant chains have discovered that improving the nutritional value of their products is good for sales. When you eat at one of these chains, choose a plain hamburger (instead of a larger one topped with a sauce), a roast beef sandwich, a skinless grilled or baked chicken sandwich, a pizza without meat, or a baked potato with low-fat toppings. Select prepared vegetable salads or items from the salad bar if one is available, and use only a small amount of low-calorie dressing. And choose skim or 1 percent milk, fruit juice, water, a small soda, or a low-fat milkshake to drink.

Some fast-food chains now publish nutritional information for their fare. Request it, and pick those items that make a positive contribution to your eating plan.

Every day, millions of children and adults in the United States eat lunch in a cafeteria. Unfortunately, some of the food served in these cafeterias is far from ideal from a health standpoint. But you can do something about it—give the food service director at your firm a copy of this book. And talk to your school principal about the food served in your child's cafeteria. Schools are places of learning, so why not educate them about the benefits of a healthful diet?

TAKING THE NEXT STEPS

You probably purchased this book because you are interested in eating better. Now, armed with facts, figures, and advice, it's time for you to put it all into action.

Improving eating habits is never easy, especially at the beginning, so begin slowly. Make your dietary changes one at a time—for example, eat more fruit or vegetables, cut back on cakes and pies, reduce the amount of meat you eat at a meal, or substitute 2 percent milk for whole milk in cereal. As you become comfortable with one change, make another. Within several months, you may very well be surprised at how close you are to meeting the *Eat for Life* guidelines.

Seek out people who have the knowledge and skills to help you to eat better. Professional nutritionists (especially registered dietitians, or RDs) can teach you as much as you want to know about healthful eating, discuss food shopping strategies and cooking techniques, suggest useful sources of information, provide recipes, and help identify restaurants where it's easy to get a delicious, nutritious meal (see Appendix B). Doctors and nurses, as well as friends or neighbors who have already begun to improve their eating habits, can also be important sources of information and support.

By reading this book, you have taken an important first step to eating for life. Now it's time to think about how you can improve your next meal. Bon appétit!

APPENDIX A
U.S. RECOMMENDED DAILY ALLOWANCES

The U.S. Recommended Daily Allowances (U.S. RDAs) are a set of values developed by the Food and Drug Administration to be used as standards for the nutritional labeling of foods and dietary supplements.

TABLE A.1 U.S. Recommended Daily Allowances (U.S. RDAs)

	Adults and Children Over 4 yrs.	Children Under 4 yrs.
Protein	65 g[a]	28 g[a]
Vitamins		
Fat soluble		
A	5,000 IU	2,500 IU
D	400 IU	400 IU
E	30 IU	10 IU
Water soluble		
C	60 mg	40 mg
Thiamin	1.5 mg	0.7 mg
Riboflavin	1.7 mg	0.8 mg
Niacin	20 mg	9.0 mg
Vitamin B_6	2.0 mg	0.7 mg
Vitamin B_{12}	6 μg	3 μg
Folacin	0.4 mg	0.2 mg
Biotin	0.3 mg	0.15 mg
Pantothenic acid	10 mg	5 mg
Minerals		
Calcium	1.0 g	0.8 g
Copper	2 mg	1 mg
Iodine	150 μg	70 μg
Iron	18 mg	10 mg
Magnesium	400 mg	200 mg
Phosphorus	1.0 g	0.8 g
Zinc	15 mg	8 mg

[a]If protein efficiency ratio of protein is equal to or better than that of casein, U.S. RDA is 45 g for adults and 20 g for children under 4 years of age.

SOURCE: U.S. Food and Drug Administration.

APPENDIX B
RESOURCES

Registered Dietitians (RDs) are uniquely qualified to assess your nutritional status and provide counseling. Many RDs are listed in the telephone Yellow Pages, or they may be contacted through the nearest hospital or health department. A list of RDs who provide consultation services can be obtained by contacting

The National Center for Nutrition and Dietetics
The American Dietetic Association
216 West Jackson Boulevard
Suite 800
Chicago, IL 60606-6995
(312) 899-4853
(800) 366-1655

The U.S. Department of Agriculture's campaign, "Eating Right . . . The Dietary Guidelines Way," provides a variety of educational materials that can be ordered at modest prices from the Consumer Information Center (Pueblo, CO 81009). The materials include

- Preparing Foods and Planning Menus Using the Dietary Guidelines
- Making Bag Lunches, Snacks, and Desserts Using the Dietary Guidelines
- Shopping for Food and Making Meals in Minutes Using the Dietary Guidelines
- Eating Better When Eating Out Using the Dietary Guidelines

One very useful cookbook is *The American Heart Association Cookbook.* It is available at most bookstores.

Information on the calorie, carbohydrate, protein, fat (including saturated and unsaturated fatty acids), sodium, vitamin, and mineral content of common foods can be found in *Nutritive Value of Foods* (Home and Garden Bulletin Number 72). This book, issued by the Department of Agriculture, can be purchased from the Superintendent of Documents, Government Printing Office (Washington, DC 20402).

APPENDIX C

COMMITTEE ON DIET AND HEALTH

ARNO G. MOTULSKY (*Chairman*), Center for Inherited Diseases, University of Washington, Seattle

EDWIN L. BIERMAN (*Vice Chairman*), Division of Metabolism, Endocrinology, and Nutrition, University of Washington School of Medicine, Seattle

DeWITT S. GOODMAN (*Vice Chairman*) (deceased), Institute of Human Nutrition, Columbia University, New York

DONALD B. McCORMICK (*Vice Chairman*), Department of Biochemistry, Emory University School of Medicine, Atlanta, Georgia

CLAUDE D. ARNAUD, JR., Program in Osteoporosis and Bone Biology, University of California, San Francisco

JOHN C. BAILAR III, Department of Epidemiology and Biostatistics, McGill University School of Medicine, Montreal, Quebec, Canada

HENRY BLACKBURN, Division of Epidemiology, School of Public Health, University of Minnesota, Minneapolis
GEORGE A. BRAY, Section of Diabetes and Clinical Nutrition, University of Southern California, Los Angeles
KENNETH K. CARROLL, Biochemistry Department, University of Western Ontario, London, Ontario, Canada
GEOFFREY R. HOWE, National Cancer Institute of Canada Epidemiology Unit, Faculty of Medicine, University of Toronto, Toronto, Ontario, Canada
LUCILLE S. HURLEY (deceased), Department of Nutrition, University of California, Davis
LAURENCE N. KOLONEL, Cancer Research Center of Hawaii, University of Hawaii, Honolulu
HENRY C. McGILL, JR., Southwest Foundation for Biomedical Research, University of Texas Health Science Center, San Antonio
ANTHONY B. MILLER, Department of Preventive Medicine and Biostatistics, University of Toronto, Toronto, Ontario, Canada
LOT B. PAGE, National Institute on Aging, Bethesda, Maryland
RICHARD M. SCHIEKEN, Division of Pediatric Cardiology, Medical College of Virginia East Hospital, Richmond
RICHARD B. SHEKELLE, School of Public Health, University of Texas Health Science Center, Houston
LOUIS TOBIAN, JR., Hypertension Section, University of Minnesota Hospital School of Medicine, Minneapolis
ELEANOR R. WILLIAMS, Department of Human Nutrition and Food Systems, University of Maryland, College Park

Adviser

PAUL D. STOLLEY, Department of Medicine, University of Pennsylvania, Philadelphia

Food and Nutrition Board Liaison

WILLIAM E. CONNOR, Department of Medicine, Oregon Health Sciences University, Portland

M.R.C. GREENWOOD, Department of Biology, Vassar College, Poughkeepsie, New York

Food and Nutrition Board Staff

SUSHMA PALMER, *Director*
FRANCES M. PETER, *Deputy Director and Editor*
CHRISTOPHER P. HOWSON, *Project Director*
FARID E. AHMED, *Project Coordinator*
SUSAN E. BERKOW, *Program Officer*
ALDON GRIFFIS, *Research Assistant*
MARIAN F. MILLSTONE, *Research Assistant*
AVIS I. HARRIS, *Senior Secretary*
DOROTHY MAJEWSKI, *Senior Secretary* (until October 1988)
MICHELLE E. SMITH, *Senior Secretary* (from November 1988)
ELSIE C. STURGIS, *Senior Secretary*

FOOD AND NUTRITION BOARD

M.R.C. GREENWOOD (*Chair*), University of California, Davis

DONALD B. McCORMICK (*Vice Chairman*), Department of Biochemistry, Emory University School of Medicine, Atlanta, Georgia

DeWITT S. GOODMAN (*Vice Chairman*) (deceased), Institute of Human Nutrition, Columbia University, New York

EDWIN L. BIERMAN, Division of Metabolism, Endocrinology, and Nutrition, University of Washington School of Medicine, Seattle

EDWARD J. CALABRESE, Environmental Health Program, Division of Public Health, University of Massachusetts, Amherst

JOHANNA T. DWYER, Frances Stern Nutrition Center, Boston, Massachusetts
JOHN W. ERDMAN, JR., Division of Nutritional Sciences, University of Illinois, Urbana
CUTBERTO GARZA, Division of Nutritional Sciences, Cornell University, Ithaca, New York
RICHARD J. HAVEL, Cardiovascular Research Institute, University of California School of Medicine, San Francisco
JANET C. KING, Department of Nutritional Sciences, University of California, Berkeley
JOHN E. KINSELLA, College of Agricultural and Environmental Sciences, University of California, Davis
LAURENCE N. KOLONEL, Cancer Research Center of Hawaii, University of Hawaii, Honolulu
WALTER MERTZ, Human Nutrition Research Center, Agricultural Research Service, U.S. Department of Agriculture, Beltsville, Maryland
MALDEN C. NESHEIM, Cornell University, Ithaca, New York
ARNO G. MOTULSKY (*Ex Officio*), University of Washington, Seattle
ROY M. PITKIN (*Ex Officio*), Department of Obstetrics and Gynecology, School of Medicine, University of California, Los Angeles
STEVE L. TAYLOR (*Ex Officio*), Department of Food Science and Technology, University of Nebraska, Lincoln

Executive Office Staff

CATHERINE E. WOTEKI, Director
MARCIA LEWIS, Administrative Assistant

INDEX

A

Adolescents, *see* Teenagers
Aflatoxin, 3, 130
Age
  and body mass index, 72
  and caloric intake, 80
  and gallstones, 83
  and heart disease, 99
  and weight for height, 73
Alcohol consumption
  blood alcohol levels, 124
  calories from, 36, 37, 121
  and cancer, 14, 114, 115, 125–126
  and cigarette smoking, 125
  classification of drinkers, 123–124
  deaths from, 58
  dietary guidelines, 6, 13–14, 19, 21, 23
  and heart disease, 14, 126
  and high blood pressure, 14, 65, 126
  and liver disease, 14, 77, 114, 124–125
  and nervous system diseases, 14, 126–127
  and nutritional deficiencies, 14
  and obesity, 126
  physiological effects of, 124
  during pregnancy, 14, 127
  and stroke, 126
Alcoholism, 14, 77, 114, 125
Alginates, 40
American Academy of Pediatric Dentistry, 116
American Academy of Pediatrics, 116
American Cancer Society, 20–21
American Dental Association, 16, 116
American Diabetes Association, 17, 20–21
American Dietetic Association, 15, 22, 161
American Heart Association, 17, 20–21
American Institute of Nutrition, 15
American Society for Clinical Nutrition, 15
Amino acids
  B vitamins and, 49
  essential, 29, 47
  sources, 12–13, 47
  supplements, 15
Anemia (iron deficiency), 58, 116–117
Aneurysms, 63
Angina pectoris, 62

Antioxidants, 48, 52
Artificial sweeteners, 21, 122, 129
Ascorbic acid, *see* Vitamin C
Aspartame, 129
Atherosclerosis
  cholesterol and, 61, 89
  deaths, 58, 59
  diabetes and, 69
  fat intake and, 11, 60
  mechanisms, 60–61
  and peripheral artery disease, 63
  prevention, 12, 61
  reversal, 61
  saturated fatty acids and, 92–93
  and stroke, 60, 61, 64
  vitamin C and, 111–112
  in young adults, 99
Avocado, 41, 135, 136

B

B vitamins, *see specific vitamins*
Bacon, 142
Baking soda, 52, 119
Bananas, 137
Beans
  caloric intake trends, 55
  carbohydrates in, 40
  fiber in, 41
  minerals in, 51–52
  protein in, 29, 47
  recommendations, 138
  vitamins in, 48–49
Beef fat, 45
Beer, 6, 13, 122
Beta-carotene, 110, 111
BHA and BHT, 130
Bile, 76
Bile duct cancer, 84
Biotin, 30, 50, 159
Blacks
  coronary heart disease, 63
  high blood pressure, 66, 67
  stroke, 12, 64
Bladder cancer, 68, 111, 127–128, 129
Blindness, 69
Blood
  clotting, 47, 48
  pressure, 65–66; *see also* High blood pressure
Body fat distribution
  and blood pressure, 83
  and diabetes, 70, 73
  genetic factor in, 82
  and heart disease, 73
  and stroke, 71–72
  waist-to-hip ratio, 73–74, 83
Body mass index, 71–72
Bone
  composition, 75
  formation and growth, 48, 51, 52
  mass, 15, 51, 115
Bran, 30, 40, 41, 106, 107
Bread, 91
  carbohydrates in, 137
  fiber in, 30, 41
  minerals in, 51
  protein in, 29
  recommendations, 6, 7, 12, 101, 133, 137
  vitamins in, 49, 50
Breakfast, 54–55, 153
Breakfast cereals, 48, 49
Breast cancer, 2, 11, 24, 68, 84, 96, 97, 113, 125
Breast milk, 98–99
Breastfeeding, 15
Brewer's yeast, 51
Broccoli, 48
Butter
  cholesterol in, 55
  fats in, 27, 28, 41, 42, 45, 134, 143
  margarine substituted for, 132–133
  and serum cholesterol, 92
  vitamins in, 48, 110

C

Cabbage, 48
Cafeteria food, 154
Caffeine, 112, 127, 128
Cakes and cookies, 28, 41, 149
Calcium
  and chronic disease, 115–116
  dietary guidelines, 6, 15, 21, 23
  and osteoporosis, 15, 23, 115
  plaque formation in blood stream, 60
  protein intake and, 11, 103
  recommended intake, 115, 159
  role in the body, 30, 50, 51, 115

sources, 15, 23, 51, 115, 138
supplements, 15, 21, 115
vitamin D and, 21, 47, 48
Caloric intake
activity level and, 35–36, 54
age and, 80
from carbohydrates, 54–55
and dietary supplement use, 15
and expenditures, 35–36, 79–81
from fat, 10, 54–55
from meat and poultry, by cut, 141
and obesity, 2
from saturated fatty acids, 10, 25–26
and weight, 22, 37, 80–81
Cancer
alcohol consumption and, 113, 125–126
caloric intake and, 97
coffee and tea and, 127–128
deaths, 58, 59, 67
diagnosis, 68
diet-related types, 68
fats and, 2, 4, 11, 87, 96–97, 128
fiber and, 106
mechanisms in, 67–68, 125–126
preventive foods and nutrients, 12, 97, 110–111
protein and, 102
rates, 67
recommendations for risk reduction, 17, 20–21, 25
risk of, 27, 69
saturated fatty acids and, 4, 97
vitamin A and, 110–111
vitamin E and, 113
weight and, 84, 97
see also specific kinds of cancer
Canola oil, 43, 94, 133, 142, 143
Carbohydrates
caloric content, 36, 37
consumption trends, 54–55
defined, 29–30
dental caries and, 77, 103–104
fattening foods, 101, 133
and heart disease, 101
metabolism, 38, 48, 49, 51
and noninsulin-dependent diabetes, 104
role in the body, 34
sources, 38
structure, 39
types, *see* Complex carbohydrates; Fiber; Sugars
Carotenoids, 48, 110, 137
Carrageenan, 40
Carrots, 12
Cavities, *see* Dental Caries
Cellulose, 30, 40–41
Cereals
carbohydrates in, 29, 40, 137
fiber in, 30, 41
food additives in, 129, 130
malted, 40
minerals in, 51–52
protein in, 47
recommended intakes, 6, 11, 12, 132, 133
vitamins in, 48–49
whole-grain, 30, 133
see also Grains and grain products
Cerebral hemorrhage, 64; *see also* Stroke
Cerebral thrombosis, 64; *see also* Stroke
Cervical cancer, 84, 111
Cheeses, 52, 92, 104, 132, 135, 138
Chest pain, 62
Chewing tobacco, 113–114
Children
calcium intake, 115
eating habits, 99
fat intake, 11, 81, 98–99
fluoride supplements, 16, 117
iron intake, 19
Chloride, 31, 51
Chocolate, 28, 41
Cholesterol (dietary)
children's intake, 99
consumption trends, 55
guidelines, 6, 10, 11, 18, 20, 22
responsiveness to, 93
and serum cholesterol, 10, 93
sources, 10, 28, 45, 46, 55, 141, 142, 149
Cholesterol (serum)
cholesterol intake and, 10, 93
coffee drinking and, 128
defined, 28
desirable levels, 46
diagnosis, 24
fiber intake and, 105–106
and heart disease, 25–27, 60, 87–91

high, prevalence of, 60
protein intake and, 102
role in the body, 28, 45, 76, 84
saturated fatty acids and, 10, 25–26, 95, 102
structure, 46
studies monitoring health effects, 89
total, 28, 46
types, 46
vitamin C and, 112
weight and production of, 84
see also HDL cholesterol; LDL cholesterol

Chromium, 30, 51
Cigarette smoking, 63, 81–82, 96, 125, 128
Cirrhosis of the liver, 58, 59, 76–77, 124–125
Citrus fruits, 12, 48, 57, 137
Cobalamin, *see* Vitamin B_{12}
Cobalt, 30
Cocktails, 6, 13
Cocoa butter, 92, 143
Coconut, 41, 44, 136
Coconut oil, 10, 142, 143, 146
Coffee and tea, 127–128
Colon cancer, 2, 11, 12, 68, 84, 96, 106, 128
Colorectal cancer, 68, 97
Complex carbohydrates
defined, 29–30
and dental caries, 103–104
dietary guidelines, 12, 19, 21, 22
food supply, 55
high-fat, 137
protective effects of, 103–104
role in the body, 41
serving recommendations, 6, 11, 12, 22, 134
sources, 22, 132, 135, 138
structure, 39
types, 39
see also Fiber; Starches

Congestive heart failure, 77
Connective tissue growth, 48
Cookbooks, 162
Cooking, 21
broiling, 148
frying, 133, 147
microwaving, 148
salt addition during, 14
sauteing, 148
sodium equivalent, 14
steaming, 147
stir-frying, 147–148
substitutions, 149–152
vitamin destruction during, 48

Copper, 30, 48, 50, 51, 159
Corn oil, 143
Corn syrups, 40, 144
Coronary heart disease, 2, 13, 24–25, 27, 62, 73, 85
Cottage cheese, 138–139
Cottonseed oil, 143
Couch potatoes, energy needs, 36
Council on Scientific Affairs, dietary recommendation to U.S. public, 18–19
Crackers, 135, 145–146
Cream cheese, 150

D

Dairy products
cholesterol in, 10, 28, 46
fats in, 10, 28, 41, 102, 135, 138
low-fat/nonfat, 11, 132, 138–139
minerals in, 51–52, 115, 138
protein in, 47, 102
shopping for, 138–139
substitutes for, 150
see also specific products

Dark-green vegetables, 15, 48, 49, 51, 110
Deficiency diseases, 1–2, 55, 57–58
Dementia, 126
Dental caries, 2, 16, 58, 59, 77, 116
Desserts, 130, 135, 136
Dextrose, 144
Diabetes mellitus
body fat distribution and, 70, 73
complications of, 69, 104
deaths, 58, 59
insulin-dependent, 69–70
mechanisms in, 69
recommendations for risk reduction, 20–21
treatment, 69–70
types, 69–70
weight and, 83
see also Noninsulin-dependent diabetes mellitus

Diet, changes over time, 53–56

Dietary guidelines
alcoholic beverages, 6, 13–14, 19, 21
calcium, 6, 15
cholesterol, 6, 10, 11, 18, 20, 22
complex carbohydrates, 6, 12, 19, 21, 22
conflicts in, 23
development of, 3–5
exercise, 6, 13, 18, 20
fat, 6, 10–11, 18, 20, 22
fiber, 19, 21, 22–23
fluoride, 6, 16
of other expert groups, 16–23; *see also specific groups*
polyunsaturated fatty acids, 18, 20
protein, 6, 12–13, 23
risk-reducing, for specific diseases, 20–21, 24–27
salt (sodium chloride), 6, 14, 19, 21
saturated fatty acids, 6, 10–11, 18, 20, 22
sugars (simple), 18, 20
vitamin/mineral supplements, 6, 15–16
see also specific foods
Dietary terms/definitions
carbohydrates, 29–30
cholesterol, 28
fats, 27–28
fatty acids, 28
minerals, 30–31
protein, 28–29
vitamins, 30
Dieting, 5–7, 84–85
Dietitians, 161
Disaccharides, 39; *see also* Sugars
Drinking water, fluoride in, 16, 19, 51, 116

E

Eating out, 4–5, 55, 152–154
Eating patterns
changes in, 55, 154–155
dieting, 5–7
guidelines, *see* Dietary guidelines
Education/information
materials, 161–162
programs, 3, 4
Eggs
cholesterol in, 10, 28, 46, 55, 149
consumption trends, 55
limiting intakes, 11
minerals in, 51, 52
role in cooking, 149
substitutes for, 132, 149–150
vitamins in, 48, 49, 110
Eicosapentaenoic acid, 44, 45
Electrolytes, 31, 50
Endometrial cancer, 13, 68, 84, 97
Energy, *see* Caloric intake; Food energy
Enzymes, 46, 47
Esophageal cancer, 2, 68, 111, 113–114, 125
Ethanol, *see* Alcohol consumption; Alcoholism
Ethnic cuisine, 5, 91–92, 153
Exercise
bicycle riding, 36
and blood pressure, 96
caloric intake and, 35, 54
guidelines, 6, 13, 17, 18, 20, 22
and weight, 13, 37, 81

F

Familial hypercholesterolemia, 90–91
Family history of disease, and prevention, 24
Fast food, 4–5, 154
Fat-soluble vitamins, 30, 47–50, 159; *see also specific vitamins*
Fats (dietary)
caloric intake from, 10, 36, 37, 54–55
and cancer, 2, 4, 11, 87, 96–97, 128
and children's health, 98–99
consumption trends, 53, 54–55
defined, 27–28
dietary guidelines, 6, 10–11, 18, 20, 22
energy conversion from, 37
and gallstones, 98
and heart disease, 2, 4, 11, 87, 88
hidden, in foods, 134–135
and high blood pressure, 95–96
metabolism of, 51
role in the body, 34, 37, 41
solubility, 41–42
sources, 27–28, 41, 141
substitution of leaner foods for, 11
structure, 41
see also Fatty acids; Triglycerides

Fatty acids
  defined, 28
  essential, 11, 43–44
  and heart disease, 60, 91–94
  niacin and, 49
  structure, 42–43
  see also Monounsaturated fatty acids; Polyunsaturated fatty acids; Saturated fatty acids; *and specific fatty acids*
Fetal alcohol syndrome, 127
Fiber (dietary)
  and cancer, 106
  guidelines, 19, 21, 22–23
  and heart disease, 105–106
  and mineral deficiency, 107
  protective effects of, 30, 103, 105, 106, 107
  role in the body, 41
  and serum cholesterol, 105–106
  sources, 12, 22, 40–41, 105, 107, 138
  supplements, 21, 107
  types of, 105
Fish
  cholesterol in, 10
  consumption trends, 55
  cooking, 148
  minerals in, 51, 52
  protein in, 140, 142
  recommended intake, 19
  substitution for meats, 11, 19, 140, 142
  vitamins in, 48, 49
Fish oils, 44
Fluoride, 30
  and dental caries, 116
  dietary guidelines, 6, 16, 19
  role in the body, 51
  sources, 51, 116
  supplements, 16, 117
Folacin, 30, 49, 114, 159
Food additives, 19, 40, 128–130
Food energy
  availability of, 54
  best sources, 29, 40
  from carbohydrates, 49
  dieting and efficiency of conversion, 85
  from fats, 41, 49
  measure of, 35; *see also* Caloric intake
  nutrients aiding conversion of, 48, 49, 51, 52
  from protein, 49
  requirements, 35, 36
  role in the body, 35
  storage as fat, 81
Food industry, recommended changes for, 4–5
Food labels
  fat types, 146
  on frozen foods, 146–147
  health claims, 136, 139, 144
  ingredient lists, 144, 146
  nutrition information, 144–145, 146
  serving size, 145–146
  vitamin/mineral information, 110, 146
Food processing, 4, 40; *see also* Cooking
Food shopping
  dairy products, 138–139
  frozen food, 146–147
  fruits and vegetables, 136–137
  grain products, 137
  legumes, 138
  meats and poultry, 139–140, 141
  packaged foods, 144–146
  packaged meats, 142–144
  seafood, 140, 142
  vegetable oils, 142
Food supply, changes in, 53–55
Foods
  contaminants in, 122, 130
  guidelines for choosing, 132–133, 162
  menu planning, 33–34, 133–136
  preparation, *see* Cooking
  see also Food processing; Food shopping; *and specific foods*
Fried foods, 11, 133
Frozen foods, shopping for, 142–146
Fructose, 29, 39, 40, 103, 144
Fruits and vegetables
  energy conversion from, 39
  nutrients in, 28, 30, 31, 40, 41, 48, 49, 51, 52, 105, 118, 133
  preparation, 130, 147–148
  serving recommendations, 5, 6, 7, 11, 12, 22, 134, 135
  shopping for, 136–137

G

Galactose, 40
Gallbladder cancer, 84

Gallbladder disease, 13
Gallstones
 age and, 83
 fat intake and, 98
 fiber intake and, 106
 obesity and, 76, 83, 98
 prevalence, 58, 59
 weight and, 83–84
Gangrene, 63, 69
Genetic factors in chronic disease, 25, 65, 82
Genetic material, production aids, 49
Glucose, 29, 39, 69, 83
Goiter, 1, 58
Grains and grain products
 aflatoxin contamination, 3
 consumption trends, 55
 nutrients in, 40, 48, 49, 51, 52, 105
 recommendations, 22
 shopping for, 137–138
 see also Cereals
Green peppers, 48
Green vegetables, 12, 48, 49, 51
Growth, 48
Guidelines, *see* Dietary guidelines
Guar gum, 40, 106, 107
Gums, 40

H

Hardening of the arteries, *see* Atherosclerosis
HDL cholesterol, 28, 46, 61, 90, 91, 94
Heart attack, 4
 alcoholic beverages and, 126
 cause, 10, 62
 cholesterol and, 88, 90, 93
 deaths from, 63
 diabetes and, 69
 fiber and, 106
 protein and, 102
 risk reduction, 93, 106, 126
 saturated fatty acids and, 88, 95
Heart disease
 alcohol consumption and, 14, 126
 carbohydrates and, 101
 coffee and tea and, 128
 deaths, 58, 59
 fats and, 2, 4, 60, 87, 88
 fatty acids and, 60, 91–94
 fiber and, 105–106
 geographic differences in incidence, 88–89
 potassium and, 118
 protective foods and nutrients, 13, 23, 126
 protein and, 102
 recommendations for risk reduction, 17, 20–21
 salt intake and, 25
 saturated fatty acids and, 4, 25–26, 94–95
 serum cholesterol and, 25–27, 87–91
 and stroke, 60
 weight and, 82
 see also Atherosclerosis
Height/weight tables, 17, 71, 73, 74
Hemachromatosis, 76
Hemicellulose, 40, 41
High blood pressure
 alcohol consumption and, 14, 65, 126
 body fat distribution and, 83
 diagnosis/detection, 24, 66–67
 effects on body systems, 65
 fats and, 95–96
 fiber intake and, 106
 kidney disease and, 65
 obesity and, 65
 potassium and, 118
 prevalence, 14, 58–59, 66–67
 salt and, 2, 25, 65, 118
 and stroke, 64
 symptoms, 65–66
 weight and, 13, 65, 82–83
High blood sugar, 40
High-density lipoproteins, 28; *see also* HDL cholesterol
High-fructose corn syrups, 40, 144
Honey, 39, 144
Hot dogs, 142, 144
Hypertension, *see* High blood pressure

I

Ice cream, 36, 37, 38, 132
Ice milk, 36, 37, 38
Infants and toddlers
 dietary recommendations, 15, 25, 98
Insulin, 51

Inter-Society Commission for Heart Disease Resources, 20–21
Iodine, 1, 30, 51, 58, 159
Ions, 50, 52
Iron, 30, 50, 51
  absorption, 50, 51
  deficiency, 58, 116–117
  dietary recommendations, 11, 19
  U.S. RDAs, 159
  role in the body, 51, 116–117
  sources, 51, 116
Italian food, 91–92, 153

K

Kidney disease, 65, 69

L

Labels, *see* Food labels
Lactose, 29, 39, 40
Lard, 27, 28, 41, 132–133, 143, 146
Laryngeal cancer, 111, 125
Lauric acid, 42, 92
LDL cholesterol
  coffee drinking and, 128
  defined, 28, 46
  dietary cholesterol and, 93
  in familial hypercholesterolemia, 90–91
  fiber intake and, 106
  and heart attack, 90
  role in the body, 61, 90
  saturated fatty acid intake and, 92, 94
  typical values, 90
  vegetable oils and, 94, 133, 146
Lecithin, 15
Legumes, 6, 11, 12, 19, 22, 105, 132, 137–138; *see also specific legumes*
Lentils, 138
Lettuce, 136
Lignin, 40, 41
Linoleic acid, 42, 43–44
Linolenic acid, 42, 43, 96
Lipids, *see* Cholesterol; Fats; Fatty acids
Lipoproteins, 46, 90; *see also* High-density lipoproteins; Low-density lipoproteins
Liver (food), 46, 48, 49, 51, 68, 110
Liver cancer, 125, 130
Liver disease
  alcohol consumption and, 14, 114, 125–126
  deaths, 58, 59
  see also Cirrhosis of the liver
Locust bean gum, 40
Low-density lipoproteins, 28; *see also* LDL cholesterol
Lunch meats, 142
Lung cancer, 12, 68, 110–111, 113

M

Macrominerals, 50; *see also* Calcium; Phosphorus
Magnesium, 51, 159
Maltose, 39–40, 144
Manganese, 30, 51
Maple syrup, 39, 144
Margarine, 27, 41, 44, 132–133, 139, 143
Meats and poultry
  caloric content, 37, 141
  cholesterol, 28, 46, 140, 141
  consumption trends, 53–55, 92
  cured, 129
  fats in, 10, 28, 41, 102, 141
  grades, 140
  lean, 4, 11, 53, 132, 139–140, 150–151
  minerals in, 31, 51, 52
  packaged, 142–144
  portion sizes, 11, 13, 135, 140
  preservatives, 129
  protein in, 47, 102
  recommended intakes, 19, 134, 135
  saturated fatty acids, 141
  shopping for, 139–140, 142–144
  substitutes for, 132, 151–152
  vitamins in, 48, 49
Melons, 48
Men
  caloric intake and expenditure, 35–36, 80
  coronary heart disease, 63
Menu planning, 33–34, 133–136
Milk and milk products
  aflatoxin in, 3
  calories, 36, 37, 38
  carbohydrates, 38, 40

fat in, 37, 38, 45, 132, 135
fortification, 58
ice milk, 36, 37, 38
infant formula, 98–99
low-fat/nonfat, 15, 139, 147
minerals in, 15, 23, 51, 52, 132
protein in, 132
vitamins in, 48, 49, 110
see also Breast milk; Dairy products
Minerals
deficiencies, 107, 109
defined, 30–31
role in the body, 30–31, 34, 50–52
sources, 51, 52
toxicity, 114
U.S. RDAs, 159
see also Trace elements; *and specific minerals*
Molasses, 39, 144
Molybdenum, 30, 52
Monosaccharides, 39; *see also* Sugars
Monosodium glutamate, 119
Monounsaturated fatty acids
caloric intake from, 54–55
and heart disease, 95
and serum cholesterol, 94, 133
sources, 28, 43, 44, 133, 142, 143
structure, 43
Mucilage, 40
Muscle function, 51, 52, 63
Mustard greens, 137
Myocardial infarction, *see* Heart attack
Myristic acid, 42, 92

N

National Cancer Institute, 17, 20–21
National Center for Nutrition and Dietetics, 161
National Council Against Health Fraud, 15
National Institutes of Health, 20–21
National Research Council, dietary recommendations, 18–21
Native Americans, 76
Nerve function, 51, 52
Nervous system diseases, alcohol consumption and, 14, 126–127
Niacin, 1, 30, 49, 58, 114, 159
Nitrites, 129
Nitrosamines, 129
Nondairy coffee whiteners, 150
Noninsulin-dependent diabetes mellitus
body fat distribution and, 70, 83
caloric intake and, 2
carbohydrates and, 104
dietary recommendations for preventing, 17
fiber intake and, 106
obesity and, 70
risk factors, 70, 104
weight and, 13, 83
Nutrients
caloric content of, 35–37
deficiencies, 1, 14
see also specific nutrients
Nutrition counseling, 154, 161
Nuts
consumption trends, 55
fats in, 28
fiber in, 41
minerals in, 51, 52
protein in, 47
vitamins in, 48, 49

O

Oat bran, 40, 106
Oatmeal, 137
Obesity
alcohol consumption and, 126
caloric intake and, 2
and cancer, 97
and chronic disease, 17
defined, 70, 82
and gallstones, 76, 83
genetic factor, 82
and high blood pressure, 65
prevalence, 58–59, 75
Oils and fats, 11; *see also* Vegetable oils
Oleic acid, 42, 43, 45
Olive oil, 43, 45, 92, 94, 142, 143
Oral cancer, 111, 125
Orange vegetables, 48, 110
Oriental food, 153
Osteoarthritis, 13
Osteomalacia, 112–113
Osteoporosis
and bone fracture, 75, 115
calcium and, 15, 23, 115–116

and estrogen therapy, 115
prevalence, 58, 59
protein and, 102
recommendations for risk reduction, 20–21
vitamin D and, 112, 113
Ovarian cancer, 68, 84
Overweight, 70, 71, 74–75, 82, 83, 85

P

Packaged foods, shopping for, 142–146
Palm-kernel oil, 10, 143
Palm oil, 10, 44, 143
Palmitic acid, 42, 43, 92
Pancreatic cancer, 68
Pantothenic acid, 30, 49, 159
Pasta, 7, 91, 137
Peanut butter, 29
Peanut oil, 43, 142, 143
Peanuts, 3, 31
Peas, 29, 41, 138
Pectin, 30, 40, 106
Pellagra, 1, 58, 109
Peripheral artery disease, 61, 63
Phenylketonuria, 129
Phosphorus, 48, 50, 52, 102, 159
Pickled foods, 129
Pinto beans, 40
Pizza, 135
Plaque, 10
Polysaccharides, *see* Complex carbohydrates
Polyunsaturated fatty acids
and blood pressure, 96
caloric intake from, 54–55, 96
dietary guidelines, 18, 20
and heart disease, 95
omega-3, 44, 45, 142
omega-6, 44
and serum cholesterol, 95
sources, 28, 44, 142, 143
structure, 43–44
Polyvinyl chloride, 128
Popcorn, 135
Potassium, 12, 31, 52, 118, 137
Potatoes, 7, 29, 31, 40, 101, 130, 133, 137
Poultry, *see* Meats and poultry
Pregnancy
and alcohol consumption, 13, 14, 127
and coffee and tea consumption, 128
dietary supplements during, 15
Preservatives, 119, 129, 130
Processed foods, 19, 135
Prostate cancer, 2, 11, 68, 84, 97
Protein
and calcium loss, 103
caloric intake from, 36, 37, 53, 54, 55
and cancer, 102
complementary proteins, 29
complete proteins, 29
defined, 28–29
dietary guidelines, 6, 12–13, 21, 23
energy conversion from, 37
and heart disease, 102
and osteoporosis, 103
role in the body, 34, 46
and saturated fatty acids intakes, 101
and serum cholesterol, 102
sources, 29, 47, 102, 132, 138, 140, 142
structure, 47
supplements, 15, 21
U.S. RDA, 159
Pyridoxine, *see* Vitamin B_6

R

Reproduction, 48
Restaurants, 152–153
Retinoids, 110, 111
Retinol, *see* Vitamin A
Riboflavin, 30, 49, 113, 159
Rice, 29, 137
Rice bran, 40
Rickets, 58, 109, 112–113
Roughage, *see* Fiber

S

Saccharine, 129
Safflower oil, 143
Salad bars, 153–154
Salad dressings, 133, 134, 144, 150
Salt (sodium chloride)
added at the table, 133
and cancer, 14
components, 50, 52
dietary guidelines, 6, 14, 19, 21

and hypertension, 2, 25, 65, 118–119
iodized, 58
in processed foods, 4
sensitivity, 119
substitutes for, 151
Salts, 50, 52
Saturated fatty acids
and blood pressure, 96
caloric intake from, 10, 25–26, 54–55
and cancer, 4, 97
children's intake, 99
dietary guidelines, 5, 10–11, 18, 20, 22
and heart disease, 4, 11, 94–95
and serum cholesterol, 10, 25–26, 92, 94, 102
sources, 10, 23, 28, 101, 130, 132, 136, 138, 139, 141, 142, 143, 146
structure, 42
types, 42
see also specific saturated fatty acids
Sausage, 142
Scurvy, 57–58
Seafood, 44, 51, 52, 53, 135, 140, 142
Seeds, 48, 52, 55
Selenium, 30, 52, 113
Sesame oil, 143
Shellfish, 28, 46, 51, 52, 142
Shopping, *see* Food shopping
Shortening, 27–28, 41, 42, 44, 130, 146
Skin, 48, 51
Smoked foods, 129
Snacks/snacking, 55, 135
Sodium
and high blood pressure, 118–119
role in the body, 52
salt equivalent, 14
sources, 31, 52, 119
and stroke, 12
Sodium chloride, *see* Salt
Soft drinks, 40, 104, 129
Soups, 144, 150–151
Soy sauce, 135
Soybean oil, 143, 146
Soybeans, 102
Spaghetti sauce, 144
Spicy foods, 150
Spinach, 136–137
Squash, 137
Starches, 6, 29, 40, 55; *see also* Complex carbohydrates
Steak sauce, 135
Stearic acid, 42, 92
Stomach cancer, 12, 14, 68, 111, 119, 129–130
Strawberries, 48
Streptococcus mutans, 77
Stroke, 64
alcohol consumption and, 126
atherosclerosis and, 60, 61, 64
body fat distribution and, 72
cholesterol and, 10
deaths, 58, 59
diabetes and, 69
potassium and, 118
risk factors and populations, 12, 27
salt intake and, 25
signs and symptoms, 64
types, 64
Sucrose, 29, 39, 40, 103
Sugars (simple)
defined, 29
and dental caries, 103
dietary guidelines, 18, 20
energy conversion from, 39
food supply, 55
replacements listed on food labels, 144
sources, 39–40
structure, 39, 40
Sulfur, 30
Sunflower oil, 143
Supplements, *see* Vitamin/mineral supplements
Sweet potatoes, 12, 137

T

Tea, 51, 127–128
Teenagers
calcium intake, 15, 19, 115
iron intake, 19
Teeth, 51; *see also* Dental Caries
Thiamin, 30, 48, 114, 127, 159
Throat cancer, 125
Tofu, 146
Tomatoes, 48
Tortillas, 51

Trace elements
  role in the body, 34
  toxicity, 30
  see also specific elements
Triglycerides, 41, 42, 90

U

U.S. Department of Agriculture, dietary recommendations, 18–19, 161–162
U.S. Department of Health, Education, and Welfare, dietary recommendations, 18–19
U.S. Department of Health and Human Services, dietary recommendations, 18–19
U.S. Recommended Daily Allowances (U.S. RDAs), 146, 159
U.S. Senate, dietary recommendations to U.S. public, 18–19
Unsaturated fatty acids
  cis and *trans* configurations, 44–45
  see also Monounsaturated fatty acids; Polyunsaturated acids

V

Vegetable oils
  cholesterol-reducing effects, 93–94
  fat content of, 143, 146
  hydrogenation, 44, 45
  nutrients in, 28, 41, 42, 48, 135, 142
Vegetables, *see* Fruits and vegetables
Vegetarians, 15, 95, 105
Very-low-density lipoproteins, 46, 90
Viral hepatitis, 76
Vision, 48
Vitamin A, 30
  activity, 110
  and cancer, 110–111
  protective effects of, 110–111
  role in the body, 48
  sources, 48, 110, 137
  toxicity, 50
  U.S. RDA, 159
Vitamin B_1, *see* Thiamin
Vitamin B_2, *see* Riboflavin
Vitamin B_6, 30, 49, 114, 159
Vitamin B_{12}, 30, 49, 50, 114, 159
Vitamin C, 30
  and cancer, 111–112
  deficiency, 57–58
  protective effects of, 111–112
  role in the body, 49
  and serum cholesterol, 112
  sources, 48, 57, 137
  supplements, 112
  U.S. RDA, 159
Vitamin D
  and calcium absorption, 21, 47, 48, 50, 116
  and cholesterol, 45
  deficiency, 58, 112–113
  manufacture in the body, 50
  and osteomalacia, 112–113
  and osteoporosis, 112, 113
  role in the body, 47, 48, 112
  sources, 48, 58
  storage in the body, 30
  supplements, 116
  toxicity, 50
  U.S. RDA, 159
Vitamin E, 30, 48, 113, 159
Vitamin K, 30, 47, 48, 50
Vitamin/mineral supplements
  calcium, 15, 21
  dietary guidelines, 6, 15–16, 21, 23
  fluoride, 16
  need for, 15, 16, 119–120
Vitamins
  and alcoholism, 114, 127
  deficiencies, 1, 109, 114, 127
  food sources, 49–50
  role in the body, 34, 47–50
  storage in the body, 49–50
  toxicity, 50, 120
  types defined, 30
  U.S. RDAs, 159
  see also specific vitamins

W

Walnut oil, 143
Water-soluble vitamins, 30, 47–50, 159; *see also specific vitamins*
Watermelon, 137
Weight
  appropriate, determining, 70–71
  caloric intake and, 22, 37, 80–81

cancer and, 13, 84
and death rates, 70
diabetes and, 13, 83, 104
dieting cycle and, 84–85
exercise and, 13, 37, 81
fat intake and, 81
fiber consumption and, 105
gallstones and, 13, 83–84, 98
heart disease and, 13, 82
high blood pressure and, 13, 82–83
recommendations, 17
see also Body mass index; Height/weight tables; Obesity; Overweight
Wheat, 52
bran, 41, 106, 107
germ, 48
Wine, 6, 13, 122
Women
bone loss, 75, 113
calcium intake, 15, 19
caloric intake and expenditure, 35–36, 80
coronary heart disease, 63
gallstones in, 76
high blood pressure, 66
iron intake, 19, 117
vitamin/mineral supplements, 15

Y

Yeast, 130
Yellow vegetables, 12, 48, 110
Yogurt, 36, 37, 38, 52, 132, 139, 146–147, 150

Z

Zinc, 30, 52, 159